Current Clinical Strategies

Handbook of Psychiatric Drugs

2004 Edition

Lawrence J. Albers, MD
Assistant Clinical Professor
Department of Psychiatry and Human Behavior
University of California, Irvine, College of Medicine

Rhoda K Hahn, MD
Clinical Professor
Department of Psychiatry and Human Behavior
University of California, Irvine, College of Medicine

Christopher Reist, MD
Associate Professor and Vice Chair
Department of Psychiatry and Human Behavior
University of California, Irvine, College of Medicine

Current Clinical Strategies Publishing
www.ccspublishing.com/ccs

Digital Book and Updates

Purchasers of this text may download the digital book and updates at the Current Clinical Strategies Publishing Web site: www.ccspublishing.com/ccs.

Current Clinical Strategies Publishing
27071 Cabot Road
Laguna Hills, California 92653-7011
Phone: 800-331-8227
Fax: 800-965-9420
Internet: www.ccspublishing.com/ccs

Indications for medications contained in this book sometimes may not be approved by the FDA. Varying degrees of empirical evidence exist for the effectiveness of medications for non- FDA approved uses. The authors have included those off-label indications where sufficient research has been completed to warrant the consideration of these agents as treatment alternatives.

Printed in USA ISBN 1929622-39-2

Contents

Dedicated to Our Parents

Antidepressants

Serotonin-Specific Reuptake Inhibitors

I. **Indications**

A. Serotonin-Specific Reuptake Inhibitors (SSRIs) are the most widely prescribed class of antidepressants. SSRIs have proven efficacy in the treatment of major depression, dysthymia, obsessive-compulsive disorder (OCD), panic disorder, bulimia nervosa, post-traumatic stress disorder, generalized anxiety disorder and social phobia (social anxiety disorder).

B. SSRIs are also effective in the treatment of bipolar depression and premenstrual dysphoric disorder. They may have some efficacy in the treatment of pain syndromes, such as migraine headaches and chronic pain. There is some evidence that they be effective in impulse control disorders. These agents have also been used to treat behavioral components of borderline personality disorder.

II. **Pharmacology**

A. SSRIs block serotonin reuptake into presynaptic nerve terminals, leading to enhanced serotonergic neurotransmission.

B. The half-life for these agents is approximately 24 hours for the parent compound. Fluoxetine, however, has a half-life of 2-4 days, and its active metabolite, norfluoxetine, has a 7-10 day half-life. Thus it takes fluoxetine over a month to reach steady-state plasma concentrations while the other SSRIs take approximately 5 days.

C. With the exception of fluvoxamine, the SSRIs are highly bound to plasma proteins. SSRIs have significantly less effect on muscarinic, histaminic, and adrenergic receptors, compared to tricyclic antidepressants (TCAs), and the SSRIs are generally better tolerated.

III. **Clinical Guidelines**

A. **Dosage:** SSRIs have the advantage of once-daily dosing. The dosage of fluoxetine, citalopram, and paroxetine is 20 mg per day; the dosage should be decreased to 10 mg per day in the elderly. The initial dose of escitalopram is 10 mg/day. Sertraline and fluvoxamine are dosed at 50 mg per day, but the dosage is decreased to 25 mg per day in elderly patients. There is no linear relationship between SSRI dose and response. For many patients, the dosage does not need to be increased.

B. **Obsessive-Compulsive Disorder and Bulimia:** Higher dosages of SSRIs, such as 60-80 mg of fluoxetine or 200-300 mg of sertraline, have been used to treat obsessive-compulsive disorder and bulimia. While high doses may be necessary in some patients, many patients will respond to standard dosing after 6-12 weeks. When greater than 40 mg a day of fluoxetine is given, the dosage should be divided into two doses to minimize side effects.

C. **Panic Disorder:** Patients with panic disorder should be started at a low dosage to prevent exacerbation of anxiety in the initial weeks of treatment. Patients should start at 12.5- 25 mg of sertraline, 5-10 mg of paroxetine, 10-20 mg of citalopram, 5-10 mg of escitalopram, and 5 mg of fluoxetine. After 1-3 weeks, the dosage may be increased gradually to standard dosages.

D. **Response Time:** SSRIs require 2-4 weeks to begin to alleviate symptoms of depression and treatment should continue for 6-8 weeks before a patient is considered treatment refractory.

E. **Plasma Levels:** There is no correlation between plasma concentrations of SSRIs and clinical efficacy. Measuring plasma levels is not clinically indicated.

F. **Safety:** SSRIs are much safer in overdose than other antidepressants such as TCAs or MAOIs.

IV. **Adverse Drug Reactions**

A. **Tolerability:** SSRIs are better tolerated than TCAs or MAOIs.

B. **Alpha-1 Blockade:** SSRIs do not produce orthostatic hypotension because they do not block alpha-1 adrenergic receptors as the tricyclic agents do.

C. **Histaminic Blockade:** SSRIs produce markedly less sedation or weight gain than TCAs or MAOIs because of minimal effect on histamine receptors.

D. **Muscarinic Blockade:** SSRIs usually do not cause dry mouth, constipation, blurred vision, and urinary retention because they have minimal effect on muscarinic cholinergic receptors.

E. **Seizures:** SSRIs have a seizure rate of approximately 0.2%, which is slightly lower than the rate for TCAs.

F. **Serotonergic Side Effects:** The side effects of SSRIs are primarily mediated by their interaction with serotonergic neurotransmission:

1. **Gastrointestinal effects,** such as nausea and diarrhea, are the most common adverse reactions. Nausea usually improves after the first few days of treatment. Giving the medication with food often alleviates the nausea.
2. **Decreased appetite** is common early in treatment because of nausea, and this problem usually improves after several days.
3. **Insomnia** may occur with any of the SSRIs, but it is more common with fluoxetine. Insomnia usually responds to treatment with trazodone 50-100 mg qhs. The SSRI should be given in the morning if insomnia occurs.
4. SSRIs are less sedating than tricyclic antidepressants, but sedation can occur with paroxetine or fluvoxamine. If sedation occurs, the medication should be given at bedtime.
5. **Headaches** occur occasionally upon initiation of treatment. In some patients, headaches are more persistent.
6. Sexual dysfunction such as decreased libido, delayed ejaculation and anorgasmia can occur, and this problem may be treated with Sildenafil (Viagra) 50-100 mg taken one hour before sex, bupropion (75-150 mg bid), buspirone (BuSpar) 5-20 mg bid-tid, mirtazapine 15-30 mg one hour before sex, nefazodone 100 mg one hour before sex or switching the antidepressant to bupropion, nefazodone or mirtazapine.
7. Serotonin syndrome, characterized by nausea, confusion, hyperthermia, autonomic instability, tremor, myoclonus, rigidity, seizures, coma and death, can occur when SSRIs are combined with MAOIs. SSRIs should not be used for 2 weeks before or after the use of an MAOI. For fluoxetine, 5-6 weeks should elapse after discontinuation because of its long half-life.

G. **Miscellaneous Side Effects:** SSRIs may also cause sweating, anxiety, dizziness, tremors, fatigue, and dry mouth.

H. **Mania:** SSRIs, like all other antidepressants, can induce mania or rapid cycling in bipolar patients.

I. **SSRI Discontinuation Syndrome**: On discontinuation, some patients may experience dizziness, lethargy, nausea, irritability, and headaches. These symptoms are usually transient and are more likely to occur with short- acting agents such as paroxetine and fluvoxamine. These symptoms can be prevented by slowly tapering the medication over several weeks when discontinuing the drug. Discontinuation of paroxetine may be complicated by cholinergic rebound symptoms, such as diarrhea.

J. **Restlessness:** An akathisia-like syndrome has been reported with fluoxetine, and it can be treated by reducing the dose of the SSRI. The agitation with this syndrome can be profound and often requires discontinuation of the medication.

K. **Teratogenic Effects:** All SSRIs are pregnancy category C. However, there is no evidence that SSRIs cause major birth defects in humans. The impact of untreated depression on the mother and fetus must be considered when determining these risk benefit decisions. Lack of treatment during pregnancy can lead to severe adverse consequences for the woman and fetus. Data on behavioral teratogenicity is limited.

L. **Breast Feeding:** SSRIs are secreted into breast milk, and mothers should not breast feed while taking an SSRI.

V. **Drug Interactions**

A. **Cytochrome P450 Enzymes:** SSRIs are competitive inhibitors of a variety of cytochrome P450 liver enzymes. This can result in elevated plasma levels of medications metabolized by these enzymes. Elevated plasma levels may lead to toxic side effects.

B. **Potential Toxicity:** An example of these interactions is the toxic side effects of the TCA, desipramine, which can be seen when it is given concomitantly with an SSRI such as fluoxetine. Desipramine is metabolized by the liver enzyme cytochrome P4502D6 (CYP2D6) and fluoxetine is a potent inhibitor of cytochrome CYP2D6. Fluoxetine can elevate plasma desipramine levels up to 400%, with subsequent increased sedation, anticholinergic effects, tremors and potential increased risk of seizures or cardiotoxicity.

C. **Substrates/Inhibitors**

1. Table 1 lists the substrates of several P450 liver enzymes, and table 2 indicates the degree of inhibition of the enzymes by each SSRI. The greater the inhibition, the greater the likelihood of a drug-drug interaction.
2. Drugs that have a narrow therapeutic index are more likely produce toxic symptoms when combined with a strong inhibitor of their metabolism. These drugs include antiarrhythmics, anticonvulsants, warfarin, and theophylline.

D. **Warfarin**: All the SSRIs can increase levels of warfarin via P450 interactions as well as competition for plasma protein binding sites. Prothrombin times should be monitored when combining these agents.

Table 1. Substrates of the P450 Enzymes

CYP1A2	Acetaminophen Amitriptyline Caffeine Clomipramine Clozapine	Haloperidol Imipramine Methadone Olanzapine Paracetamol	Tacrine Theophylline Thioridazine Thiothixene R-Warfarin
CYP2D6	Amitriptyline Amphetamine Bufaralol Clomipramine Clozapine Codeine Debrisoquine Desipramine Dextromethorphan Donepezil Encainide	Ethylmorphine Flecainide Haloperidol Imipramine Metoprolol Mexiletine MCPP Molindone Nortriptyline Perhexiline	Perphenazine Propafenone Propranolol Nortriptyline Quinidine Risperidone Sparteine Thioridazine Timolol Tramadol
CYP2C9	Diclofenac Ibuprofen Mefenamic acid	Naproxen Phenytoin Piroxicam	Tolbutamide S-Warfarin
CYP2C19	Amitriptyline Clomipramine Diazepam	Hexobarbital Imipramine Mephenytoin	Omeprazole Proguanil Propranolol
CYP3A4	Acetaminophen Alfentanil Alprazolam Amiodarone Amitriptyline Buspirone Carbamazepine Cisapride Clarithromycin Clomipramine Clonazepam Clozapine Cortisol Cyclosporine	Dapsone Disopyramide Diltiazem Donepezil Estradiol Estrogen Erythromycin Ethosuximide Felodipine Imipramine Lidocaine Loratadine Lovastatin	Midazolam Nicardipine Nifedipine Nisoldipine Omeprazole Quetiapine Quinidine Tamoxifen Testosterone Triazolam Verapamil Zolpidem

Degree of inhibition of Cytochrome P450 Enzymes by SSRIs					
	CYP1A2	CYP2C9	CYP2C19	CYP2D6	CYP3A4
Escitalopram (Lexapro)	0/+	0/+	0/+	+	0/+
Citalopram (Celexa)	0/+	0/+	0/+	+	0/+
Fluoxetine (Prozac)	0/+	++/+++	++/+++	++++	+/++
Fluvoxamine (LuVox)	++++	0/+	++++	0/+	+++
Paroxetine (Paxil)	0/+	0/+	0/+	++++	0/+
Sertraline (Zoloft)	0/+	0/+	+/++	+	0/+

Citalopram (Celexa)

Indications: Effective for a variety of depressive and anxiety disorders.
Preparations: 20 and 40 mg scored tablets.
Dosage:

Depression: 20 mg per day, usually given at bedtime. The dosage may be increased to 40 mg per day after one week. Maximum dosage is 60 mg/day and this should be reserved for treatment refractory patients who have had a 4-6 week trial at 40 mg/day.

Elderly: 10 mg per day for one week, then increase to 20 mg/day. Treatment refractory patients may require 40 mg/day after a trial of 4-6 weeks on 20 mg/day.

Half-life: 35 hr.
Adverse Drug Reactions: Cytochrome P450: Modest, but significant inhibition of the hepatic enzyme, CYP2D6, may lead to mild elevations TCAs and antiarrhythmics.
Clinical Guidelines: Of the SSRIs citalopram has low overall effects on P450 enzymes (see table 2).

Escitalopram (Lexapro)

Indications: Effective for a variety of depressive and anxiety disorders.
Preparations: 10 and 20 mg scored tablets.

Dosage:

Depression: 10 mg per day, usually given at bedtime. The dosage may be increased to 20 mg per day after one week. Maximum dosage is 30 mg/day, and this dosage should be reserved for treatment refractory patients who have had a 4-6 week trial at 20 mg/day.

Elderly: 10 mg per day. Treatment refractory patients may require 20 mg/day after a trial of 4-6 weeks on 10 mg/day.

Half-life: 30 hr.

Adverse Drug Reactions: Cytochrome P450: Modest inhibition of the hepatic enzyme, CYP2D6, may lead to mild elevations of TCAs and antiarrhythmics.

Clinical Guidelines: Compared to the SSRIs, escitalopram has low overall effects on P450 enzymes (see table 2). Compared to racemate (citalopram), escitalopram has an improved side-effect profile (less sedation and GI upset). Sexual side effects are similar.

Fluoxetine (Prozac, Sarafem, Prozac Weekly)

Indications: Effective for a variety of depressive and anxiety disorders.

Preparations: 10, 20 mg capsules; 20 mg/5 mL solution; 10 mg scored tablet; 90 mg weekly tablet.

Dosage:

Depression: 20 mg qAM is usually effective. May increase to maximum dose of 80 mg/day. Increase dose by 20 mg/day each month in partial responders. Most patients respond at a dosage between 20-40 mg/day.

Obsessive-compulsive disorder (OCD): 20 mg/day. Increase by 20 mg/day each month if needed. Treatment of OCD may require a higher dosage than depression. Maximum dose of 80 mg/day.

Panic Disorder: Begin with 5-10 mg qAM. Increase gradually over several weeks to 10-20 mg/day.

Bulimia: Begin with 20 mg qAM and increase as tolerated up to 60 mg per day over several days to weeks.

Premenstrual Dysphoric Disorder (PMDD): Begin with 20 mg q day throughout the month. May be increased up to 60 mg/day.

Elderly: 5-80 mg/day. Due to the long half-life, elderly patients require lower doses and every-other-day dosing may be used.

Half-life: 2-5 days for fluoxetine and 7-10 days for its active metabolite, norfluoxetine.

Adverse Drug Reactions

A. Fluoxetine is a potent inhibitor of the liver enzyme, cytochrome CYP2D6. Use caution when combining with a TCA or an antiarrhythmic agent. Can also elevate levels of many neuroleptic agents and lead to dystonias, **akathisia, or other extrapyramidal symptoms.**

B. **Benzodiazepines:** Inhibition of the liver enzyme, CYP3A4, can lead to moderate plasma elevations of some benzodiazepines with increased sedation and psychomotor impairment.

C. **Carbamazepine:** Inhibition of the liver enzyme, CYP3A4, can elevate carbamazepine levels moderately. Carbamazepine levels should be monitored.

D. **Phenytoin:** Modest elevations of phenytoin via inhibition of the liver enzyme CYP2C9. Phenytoin levels should be monitored.
E. **Codeine:** Inhibition of the liver enzyme, CYP2D6, prevents conversion of codeine to its active metabolite and can prevent pain reduction.
F. Fluoxetine is more likely to produce anxiety and insomnia than the other SSRIs.
G. Refer to tables 1 and 2 for other potential drug interactions.

Clinical Guidelines: Long half-life permits daily dosing and decrease withdrawal symptoms following abrupt discontinuance of medication. Relatively safe in overdose. The long half-life of fluoxetine/norfluoxetine requires waiting at least 5 weeks after discontinuation before starting an MAOI. Several weeks should also elapse before beginning nefazodone, because nefazodone's metabolite is anxiogenic and its metabolism is impaired by fluoxetine. Patients often require bid dosing above 40 mg per day. Typical dosing would be 40 mg in the morning and 20-40 mg at noon. Late afternoon doses often disrupt sleep.

Fluvoxamine (LuVox)

Indications: Effective for a variety of depressive and anxiety disorders.
Preparations: 25, 50, 100 mg scored tablets
Dosage:

Initial Dosage: 50 mg/day, then titrate to 300 mg/day maximum, over several weeks

Elderly: 25-150 mg/day

Children: 25 mg/day initially, then increase by 25 mg per week as needed to 50-200 mg/day

Half-life: 16-20 hours.
Adverse Drug Reactions:

A. **Theophylline:** Potent inhibition of the hepatic enzyme, CYP1A2, can produce toxicity in combination with theophylline and elevate plasma levels of other CYP1A2 substrates.
B. **Clozapine:** Potent inhibition of CYP1A2 can lead to markedly elevated clozapine levels with potential for seizures and hypotension.
C. **Benzodiazepines:** Significant inhibition of the hepatic enzyme, CYP3A4, can lead to elevated levels of some benzodiazepines, such as alprazolam, with subsequent increased sedation and psychomotor impairment.
D. **Beta-Blockers:** Significant inhibition of the hepatic enzyme, CYP2C19, can lead to elevated plasma concentrations of propranolol, with further reductions in heart rate and hypotension.
E. **Calcium Channel Blockers:** Inhibition of the hepatic enzyme, CYP3A4, can produce elevated levels of calcium channel blockers, such as diltiazem, with subsequent bradycardia.
F. **Methadone:** Fluvoxamine can significantly raise plasma methadone levels.
G. **Carbamazepine:** Fluvoxamine may elevate carbamazepine levels via CYP3A4 inhibition, leading to toxicity.
H. Refer to general discussion of SSRI adverse drug interactions for side effects typical to all SSRIs and tables 1 and 2 for further potential drug interactions.

Clinical Guidelines: Patients often require bid dosing at dosages above 100-200 mg per day. Many drug interactions with cytochrome P450 metabolized medications have been reported. The other SSRIs are just as effective; therefore, it is not commonly used.

Paroxetine (Paxil, Paxil CR)

Indications: Effective for a variety of depressive and anxiety disorders.
Preparations: 10, 20, 30, 40 mg tablets; (20 mg tablet is scored); 10 mg/5 ml solution; 12.5, 25, and 37.5 mg extended (continuous) release formulation
Dosage:

Depression: 10-20 mg qhs; may increase dose by 10-20 mg/day each month if partial response occurs (maximum 80 mg/day). For Paxil CR, begin at 25 mg/day and adjust upwards by 12.5 mg per week if needed to a maximum dosage of 62.5 mg/day.

Obsessive-Compulsive Disorder: 20 mg per day to start, then increase by 10-20 mg/day per month if partial response occurs (maximum 80 mg/day).

Panic Disorder: Begin with 5-10 mg qhs, then increase dose by 10 mg every 2-4 weeks as tolerated until symptoms abate, up to 40 mg/day. For Paxil CR, begin at 12.5 mg/day and increase by 12.5 mg per week as need up to a maximum dosage of 75 mg per day.

Social Anxiety Disorder: Begin with 20 mg qhs. In some patients, an initial dosage of 10 mg qhs for one week, then 20 mg qhs, may reduce side effects, especially in highly anxious patients. If clinical response is inadequate, increase the dosage by 10-20 mg/day every 4-6 weeks to a maximum dosage of 60 mg/day.

Elderly: 5-40 mg/day for immediate release and 12.5 to 50 mg per day for Paxil CR.

Half-life: 15-20 hours
Adverse Drug Reactions: Paroxetine is a potent inhibitor of the liver enzyme, CYP2D6. Use caution when combining with TCAs, or antiarrhythmics. Can also elevate levels of some neuroleptics and increase the incidence of EPS.
Clinical Guidelines: A reduction in anxiety often occurs early in treatment due to sedating properties. Paroxetine is less activating than fluoxetine and more sedating than fluoxetine or sertraline for most patients. Paroxetine should be taken at bedtime because it has sedative properties, compared to fluoxetine of sertraline. Mild anticholinergic effects (unlike other SSRIs) may occur with paroxetine, and cholinergic rebound can occur with discontinuation. Relatively safe in overdose. Patients may require bid dosing at dosages above 40 mg per day. Paxil CR at a dosage of 37.5 mg is bioequivalent to 30 mg or immediate release Paxil. Paxil CR may have a decrease in side effects such as nausea compared to immediate release paroxetine.

Sertraline (Zoloft)

Indications: Effective for a variety of depressive and anxiety disorders.
Preparations: 25, 50, 100 mg scored tablets

Dosage:

Depression: 50 mg qAM, then increase by 50 mg/day per month in patients with partial response (maximum dose of 200 mg/day)

Obsessive-Compulsive Disorder: Begin with 50 mg qAM and increase by 50 mg/day per month in partial responders to a maximum of 200-300 mg/day

Panic Disorder/PTSD: Begin with 25 mg qAM and increase dose by 25 mg every 2-4 weeks until symptoms abate, to a maximum dose of 200 mg per day. Patients with severe anxiety or sensitivity to medication may be started at 12.5 mg for the first week.

Elderly: 25-200 mg/day

Premenstrual Dysphoric Disorder (PMDD): 50 mg per day throughout the menstrual cycle or limited to the luteal phase.

Children: 25 mg/day for ages 6-12 and 50 mg/day for adolescents age 13-17.

Half-life: 24 hours for sertraline and 2-4 days for its metabolite, desmethyl-sertraline

Adverse Drug Reactions: Cytochrome P450: Modest, but significant inhibition of the hepatic enzyme, CYP2D6, may lead to mild elevations of TCAs and antiarrhythmics.

Clinical Guidelines: Sertraline is less likely to cause sedation compared to paroxetine or fluvoxamine. It is less likely to produce restlessness or insomnia compared to fluoxetine. Sertraline,escitalopram and citalopram have the lowest overall P450 enzyme effects of the SSRIs (see table 2).

References, see page 102.

Atypical Antidepressants

Atypical antidepressants are unique compounds that are chemically unrelated to the SSRIs, TCAs and MAOIs. They are indicated for depression and require the same amount of time to achieve clinical efficacy. Like other antidepressants, these agents may cause mania or rapid cycling in bipolar patients. The use of MAOIs with these agents can lead to a serotonergic syndrome, which may be characterized by nausea, confusion, hyperthermia, autonomic instability, tremor, myoclonus, rigidity, seizures, coma and death. These antidepressants are contraindicated for two weeks before or after the use of an MAOI.

Bupropion (Wellbutrin, Zyban and Wellbutrin SR)

I. **Indications**

A. Bupropion is effective in the treatment of major depression, dysthymia, and bipolar depression. Bupropion is also used for the treatment of Attention-Deficit Hyperactivity Disorder.

B. Low-dose bupropion is used adjunctively to treat the sexual dysfunction associated with SSRIs.

II. **Pharmacology**

A. Bupropion is a unicyclic aminoketone antidepressant with a half-life of 4-24 hours. It is thought to work via inhibition of norepinephrine reuptake as well as its effect on dopaminegic neurotransmission.

B. Therapeutic levels have not been established.

III. **Clinical Guidelines**

A. **Preparations:** 75 and 100 mg regular release tablets and 100,150 and 200 mg sustained release, non-scored, tablets.

B. **Dosage**

1. **Initial Dosage:** 100 mg bid, then increase to 100 tid after 4-5 days. Although bupropion has a short half-life and is recommended for tid dosing, many clinicians use bid dosing with the regular release tablets as well as the sustained release. Do not increase by more than 100 mg every 3 days.
2. **Slow Release:** Begin with 150 mg qAM for three days, then increase to 150 mg bid for SR tabs. Maximum dose of 200 mg SR tabs bid. The sustained release bid preparation improves compliance.
3. **Average Dosage:** 300 mg/day (divided doses). Do not exceed 150 mg/dose for the regular release or 200 mg/dose with sustained release, with doses at least 6 hours apart.
4. **Dosage Range:** 75-450 mg/day (max 450 mg/day)
5. **Elderly:** 75-450 mg/day

C. **Side-Effect Profile:** Bupropion has fewer side effects than TCAs and causes less sexual dysfunction than the SSRIs. It does not produce weight gain or orthostatic hypotension.

D. **Cardiac Profile:** Bupropion does not have significant effects on cardiac conduction or ventricular function and is a good choice in patients with cardiac disease, such as congestive heart failure.

IV. **Adverse Drug Reactions**

A. **Most common side effects:** Insomnia, CNS stimulation, headache, constipation, dry mouth, nausea, tremor.

B. **Anorexia/Bulimia:** Avoid bupropion in patients with anorexia or bulimia, due to possible electrolyte changes, potentiating seizures.

C. **Liver/Renal Disease:** Use caution in patients with hepatic or renal disease, due to potential elevation of plasma bupropion levels and toxicity.

D. **Pregnancy/Lactation:** Bupropion is not recommend during pregnancy or while breast feeding.

E. **Seizures:** Bupropion has a seizure rate of 0.4% at doses less than 450 mg/day and 4% at doses of 450-600 mg/day. The sustained release preparation has an incidence of 0.1% at doses up to 300 mg per day. Bupropion is contraindicated in patients with a history of seizure, brain injury or EEG abnormality, or recent history of alcohol withdrawal.

V. **Drug Interactions**

A. **Hepatically Metabolized Medications**

1. **Cimetidine** may inhibit the metabolism of bupropion and lead to elevated bupropion plasma levels and subsequent toxicity.
2. Bupropion is a significant inhibitor of **CYP2D6** and can lead to a two fold increase in maximum concentration or five fold increase in AUC of CYP2D6 substrates such as desipramine. If bupropion is added to a treatment regimen of medications metabolized by CYP2D6, the dosage of the other medications may need to be reduced. Examples would be certain tricyclic antidepressants, Type 1C antiarrhythmics and beta-blockers such as metoprolol.
3. **Carbamazepine, phenobarbital, and phenytoin** may induce the enzymes responsible for the metabolism of bupropion with a subsequent decrease in plasma bupropion levels.
4. **Dopamine Agonists:** Levodopa may cause confusion or dyskinesias.

B. **MAOIs:** Combining bupropion with an MAOI can lead to a serotonergic syndrome with severe toxicity.

Duloxetine (Cymbalta)

I. **Indications (FDA approval pending).**

A. Duloxetine is effective for the treatment of major depression.

II. **Pharmacology**

A. Duloxetine blocks serotonin and norepinephrine transporters.

B. Half life is 12 hours.

III. **Clinical Guidelines**

A. **Preparations:** 20 mg capsules.

B. **Dosage.**

1. **Initial dosage:** 20 - 60 mg po q am.
2. **Average dosage:** 60 mg po q am.

C. Small increases in heart rate can be observed.

D. Abrupt discontinuation can be associated with transient sleep disturbance and increases in HR.

IV. **Adverse Drug Reactions**
   A. **Common Adverse Reactions:** nausea, dry mouth, dizziness, constipation, headache.
V. **Drug Interactions:** Not yet determined.

Gepirone ER

I. **Indications (FDA approval pending).**
   A. Gepirone is effective in the treatment of major depression.
II. **Pharmacology**
   A. Gepirone is a pyridinyl piperazine 5HT1A agonist.
   B. Gepirone has differential action at presynaptic (agonist) and post-synaptic (partial agonist) 5-HT1A receptors. Compared to buspirone, it has much less D2 receptor affinity.
III. **Clinical Guidelines**
   A. **Preparations:** Extended-release 20 mg tablets.
   B. **Dosage**
      1. **Initial dosage:** 20 mg PO qAM, increase every 4 days by 20 mg.
      2. **Average dosage:** 60 mg/day is likely to be the most common dosage.
      3. **Dosage range:** 40-80 mg/day.
   C. Gepirone has minimal effects on weight, sexual function, or sedation.
IV. **Adverse Drug Reactions**
   A. **Common Adverse Reactions:** Dizziness, nausea, insomnia, nervousness, dry mouth, and GI distress.
V. **Drug Interactions**
   A. Gepirone does not inhibit P450 enzymes to a significant extent.
   B. Because it is metabolized through by the CYP3A4 enzyme primarily (CYP2D6 to a lesser extent), inhibitors of CYP3A4 can alter kinetics.

Nefazodone (Serzone)

I. **Indications**
   A. Nefazodone is effective in the treatment of major depression, dysthymia, and the depressed phase of bipolar disorder.
   B. Nefazodone (Serzone) is also used clinically for premenstrual dysphoric disorder, chronic pain, and posttraumatic stress disorder.
II. **Pharmacology**
   A. Nefazodone is the phenylpiperazine analog of trazodone and has a half-life of 2-18 hours. Nefazodone inhibits presynaptic serotonin reuptake and blocks postsynaptic serotonin receptors (5HT-2A).
   B. Therapeutic levels have not been established.
III. **Clinical Guidelines**
   A. **Preparations:** 50, 100, 150, 200, and 250 mg tablets; the 100 and 150 mg tablets are scored.
   B. **Dosage**
      1. **Initial dosage:** 50-100 mg bid, then increase gradually after several days to weeks by 50-100 mg per day.
      2. **Average dosage:** 300-500 mg/day with bid dosing.

3. **Dosage range:** 50-600 mg/day.
4. **Elderly:** Start with 50 mg/day, range: 100-200 bid.

C. **REM Sleep:** Nefazodone does not suppress REM sleep, unlike most antidepressants.

D. **Sexual Functioning:** Unlike other antidepressants, nefazodone has no adverse effects on sexual functioning.

IV. Adverse Drug Reactions

A. **Common Adverse Reactions:** The most common side effects are nausea, dry mouth, dizziness, sedation, agitation, constipation, weight loss, and headaches.

B. **Hepatic Disease:** Cases of life-threatening hepatic failure have been reported at a rate of 1 case of hepatic failure resulting in death or liver transplant per 250,000-300,000 patient years of nefazodone treatment. While there is no evidence that pre-existing liver disease increases the likelihood of liver failure ,nefazodone should not be initiated if active liver disease or elevated transaminases are present as it complicates monitoring. Patients who develop increased transaminases more than three times normal should be discontinued from treatment.

C. **Alpha Adrenergic Blockade:** Nefazodone produces less orthostatic hypotension than trazodone or tricyclic antidepressants.

D. **Histaminic Blockade:** Nefazodone has little effect on histamine receptors and produces less weight gain than TCAs or trazodone.

E. **Cardiac Effects:** Nefazodone does not alter cardiac conduction.

V. Drug Interactions

A. **CYP3A4:** Nefazodone is a significant inhibitor of the hepatic CYP3A4 enzyme, and levels of all medications metabolized by this enzyme may be elevated. Levels of triazolam and alprazolam may be increased.

B. **Cytochrome P450 Inhibitors:** A metabolite of nefazodone, CPP, is inactivated by the cytochrome P450 enzyme system. In the presence of a strong inhibitor hepatic CYP2D6 enzyme, such as fluoxetine, M-CPP is not broken down, resulting in anxiety. When switching from fluoxetine or paroxetine to nefazodone, a wash out period of 3-4 days for paroxetine and several weeks for fluoxetine is recommended to avoid this adverse reaction.

C. **Other Cytochrome P450 Enzymes:** Nefazodone does not appear to affect the metabolism of medications metabolized by other P450 enzymes.

D. **Digoxin:** Nefazodone can produce modest increases in digoxin levels.

E. **MAOI:** The combination of nefazodone with a MAOI can lead to a serotonergic syndrome and severe toxicity.

Trazodone (Desyrel)

I. Indications

A. Approved for use in depressive disorders. It is also used clinically to reduce anxiety and decrease agitation and aggression in elderly demented patients.

B. Trazodone is commonly prescribed for insomnia, and it is also effective in some patients with chronic pain syndromes.

II. Pharmacology

A. Trazodone is a triazolopyridine with a half-life of 4-9 hours.

B. Its efficacy is related primarily to inhibition of presynaptic serotonin reuptake, with possible mild postsynaptic serotonergic agonism.

C. Plasma levels are not clinically useful.

III. Clinical Guidelines

A. **Preparations:** 50, 100, 150, and 300 mg tablets.

B. **Dosage:**

1. **Initial dosage:** 50-100 mg qhs, then increase by 50 mg/day as tolerated. May require bid dosing initially.
2. **Average dosage:** 300-600 mg/day.
3. **Dosage range:** 200-600 mg/day.
4. **Elderly:** 50-500 mg/day.
5. **Insomnia:** 25-200 mg qhs.

C. **Tolerability:** Many patients are unable to tolerate the sedation and hypotension associated with an antidepressant dosage. This significantly limits its utility in the treatment of depression. It is therefore most often used for insomnia, especially in patients with SSRI-induced insomnia.

IV. Adverse Drug Reactions

A. **Histaminic Blockade:** Trazodone is a potent antihistamine and can lead to significant sedation and weight gain.

B. **Alpha-1 Adrenergic Blockade:** Marked Inhibition of alpha-1 adrenergic receptors often leads to severe hypotension, especially at high doses. Reflex tachycardia and dizziness may also occur.

C. **Cholinergic Blockade:** Trazodone has little impact on muscarinic receptors and does not produce the anticholinergic effects seen with TCAs.

D. **Dry Mouth**: Trazodone commonly causes dry mouth.

E. **Cardiac Effects:** Trazodone has little effect on cardiac conduction; however, there have been reports of exacerbation of arrhythmias in patients with preexisting conduction abnormalities. It should be avoided in patients with recent myocardial infarction.

F. **Priapism:** A prolonged, painful penile erection occurs in 1/6000 patients, due to alpha-2 blockade. Patients can be treated with intracavernal injection of epinephrine.

G. **Miscellaneous:** Nausea, GI irritation and headaches may occur.

H. **Pregnancy/Lactation:** Avoid use in pregnancy due to potential teratogenicity. Patients should not breast feed while using trazodone.

I. **Overdose:** Trazodone is much safer in overdose than TCAs, but fatalities can occur with combined overdose with alcohol or sedative/hypnotics.

J. **ECT:** Use of trazodone is not recommended during ETC.

V. Drug Interactions

A. **CNS Depressants:** Trazodone may potentiate the effects of other sedating medications.

B. **Fluoxetine** may elevate trazodone levels, but the combination is generally safe and low-dose trazodone is very effective in treating insomnia due to fluoxetine.

C. **Digoxin/Phenytoin:** Trazodone may elevate plasma levels of these drugs.

D. **Warfarin:** Trazodone has been reported to alter prothrombin time in patients on warfarin.

E. **MAOIs:** Avoid combining trazodone with MAOIs due to the potential of inducing a serotonergic syndrome.

Venlafaxine (Effexor and Effexor XR)

I. **Indications**

A. Venlafaxine is effective in the treatment of major depression, dysthymia,other depressive disorders and anxiety disorders such as generalized anxiety disorder.

B. It may have some efficacy in Attention-Deficit Hyperactivity Disorder as well as chronic pain management.

II. **Pharmacology**

A. Venlafaxine is a phenylethylamine. The half-life is 5 hours for venlafaxine and 10 hours for its active metabolite, O-desmethylvenlafaxine.

B. Venlafaxine is a selective inhibitor of norepinephrine and serotonin reuptake.

C. Therapeutic plasma levels have not been established.

III. **Clinical Guidelines**

A. **Preparations:** 25, 37.5, 50, 75, 100 mg scored immediate release tablets; and 37.5, 75, and 150 mg extended release capsules.

B. **Dosage**

1. **Immediate Release:** 75 mg on the first day in two or three divided doses with food. The dose may be increased upward in increments of 75 mg per day as clinically indicated with an average dose between 75 to 225 mg per day in bid dosing. Patients usually require several days on a given dosage before it can be increased.
2. **Extended Release:** Begin with 37.5 to 75 mg once a day with food, and increase the dosage gradually up to 225 mg if needed with an average dosage of 150 to 175 mg per day.
3. **Dosage range:** 75-375 mg/day.
4. **Elderly:** 75-375 mg/day.
5. **Generalized Anxiety Disorder:** Begin with 75 mg Qod of Effexor XR; some patients may need to begin with 37.5 mg Qod of Effexor XR for one week and then increase to 75 mg Qod. The dosage should then be titrated up as clinically indicated to a maximum dosage of 225 mg/day.

IV. **Adverse Drug Reactions**

A. **Common Side Effects:** Insomnia and nervousness are the most common side effects with venlafaxine. Nausea, sedation, fatigue, sweating, dizziness, headache, loss of appetite, constipation and dry mouth are also common. Some patients have difficulty tolerating the GI distress and sedation.

B. **Blood Pressure:** Elevations of supine diastolic blood pressure to greater than 90 mm Hg and by more than 10 mm Hg above baseline occur in 3-7% of patients. Blood pressure should be monitored periodically in patients on venlafaxine, especially if there is a history of hypertension.

C. **Sexual:** Abnormalities of ejaculation/orgasm occur in approximately 10% of patients.

D. **Seizures:** Seizures occur in 0.3% of patients.

E. **Discontinuation Syndrome:** Venlafaxine can produce dizziness, insomnia, dry mouth, nausea, nervousness, and sweating with abrupt discontinuation. It should be slowly tapered over several weeks when possible.

F. **Renal/Hepatic Disease:** The clearance of venlafaxine in patients with liver or renal disease is significantly altered, and the dosage should be decreased by approximately 50% in these patients.

G. **Cardiac Disease:** There is no systematic data on the use of venlafaxine in patients with recent MI or cardiac disease. It does not appear to have a significant effect on patients with normal cardiac conduction.

H. **Pregnancy/Lactation:** Avoid use in pregnant patients due to potential teratogenic effects. Breast feeding is contraindicated.

V. Drug Interactions

A. **Cytochrome P450 Interactions:** Venlafaxine does not appear to produce clinically significant inhibition of hepatic metabolism. It consequently should not significantly inhibit the metabolism of medications metabolized by these enzymes.

B. **MAOIs:** Venlafaxine should not be given concomitantly with a MAOI because of the possibility of producing a serotonergic syndrome with characteristic toxicity.

References, see page 102.

Heterocyclic Antidepressants

Tertiary Amine Tricyclic Antidepressants

I. **Indications**
   A. The heterocyclic antidepressants are used in the treatment of major depression, dysthymia, and the depressed phase of bipolar disorder.
   B. They have efficacy in anxiety disorders, such as panic disorder, social phobia, generalized anxiety disorder, and obsessive-compulsive disorder.
   C. They are useful adjuncts in the treatment of bulimia and chronic pain syndromes.

II. **Pharmacology**
   A. The heterocyclic antidepressants are postulated to work through their effects on monoamine neurotransmitters such as serotonin, norepinephrine and dopamine. These agents block the reuptake of these neurotransmitters to varying degrees and also interact with muscarinic cholinergic, alpha-1 adrenergic, and histaminic receptors which results in their characteristic side-effect profile.
   B. These antidepressants are rapidly absorbed from the gut and undergo significant first pass clearance by the liver. There is marked variability in plasma levels among individuals, which correlates with differences in cytochrome P450 isoenzymes.
   C. These medications are highly protein bound and lipid soluble. Their half-lives are usually greater than 24 hours, which allows for once-a-day dosing, and steady-state levels are reached in approximately five days.
   D. The tertiary tricyclic antidepressant amines, such as amitriptyline and imipramine, are demethylated to secondary amine metabolites, nortriptyline and desipramine, respectively. The tertiary tricyclic amines have more side effects and greater lethality in overdose because of greater blockade of cholinergic, adrenergic and histaminic receptors compared to secondary amines.

III. **Clinical Guidelines**
   A. **Choice of Drug:** The selection of a heterocyclic antidepressant should be based on a patient's past response to medication, family history of medication response, and side-effect profile. For example, if a patient has previously been effectively treated with nortriptyline, there is a good chance of a positive response if the same symptoms recur. Additionally, if a patient is sensitive to the sedative properties of medications, a secondary amine should be chosen over a tertiary amine.
   B. **Dosage:** The dosage of heterocyclic antidepressants should be titrated upward over several days to weeks to allow patients to adjust to side effects. This is a major disadvantage compared to SSRIs because it significantly increases the time to reach therapeutic effect in most patients. In general, most heterocyclics are started at a dose of 25-50 mg per day, and the daily dose is gradually increased to an average of 150-300 mg per day. Patients with anxiety disorders, such as panic disorder, should receive a lower initial dosage, such as 10 mg of imipramine. Patients with anxiety disorders may require slow titration to avoid exacerbation of anxiety

symptoms, which is common at the beginning of treatment. Anxiety and insomnia may begin to improve within a few days with these agents.

C. **Time to Response:** The most common reason for lack of response is the use of a subtherapeutic dose or lack of an adequate trial. A therapeutic trial of at least 3-4 weeks at the maximum tolerated dosage should be completed before a patient is considered a nonresponder. Some patients may require 6-8 weeks of treatment before responding.

IV. **Adverse Drug Reactions**

A. **Elderly patients** are much more sensitive to the side effects of TCAs, and they may be unable to tolerate therapeutic dosages.

B. **Anticholinergic Effects:** Cholinergic blockade can produce dry mouth, blurred vision, constipation, urinary retention, heat intolerance, tachycardia, and exacerbation of narrow angle glaucoma. Constipation may be alleviated by stool softeners. Dry mouth can be improved with the use of sugarless candy.

C. **Alpha Adrenergic Effects:** Alpha-1 adrenergic receptor blockade can lead to orthostatic hypotension, resulting in falls. Dizziness and reflex tachycardia may also occur.

D. **Histaminic Effects:** Histaminic blockade can produce sedation and weight gain. Many of these agents should be given at bedtime to prevent excess daytime sedation.

E. **Cardiotoxicity:** Heterocyclic antidepressants slow cardiac conduction, leading to intraventricular conduction delays, prolonged PR and QT intervals, AV block, and T-wave flattening. These agents are contraindicated in patients with preexisting conduction delays, such as a bundle branch block, or in patients with arrhythmias or recent myocardial infarction. These effects can also be seen with overdose. These agents can also cause tachycardia and elevations of blood pressure.

F. **Seizures:** Seizures occur at a rate of approximately 0.3%, and they are more likely to occur with elevated blood plasma levels, especially with clomipramine, amoxapine, and maprotiline.

G. **Neurotoxicity:** Heterocyclics may produce tremors and ataxia. In overdose, agitation, delirium, seizures, coma and death may occur.

H. **Serotonergic Effects:** Erectile and ejaculatory dysfunction may occur in males, and anorgasmia may occur in females.

I. **Overdose:** Heterocyclic agents are extremely toxic in overdose. Overdose with as little as 1-2 grams may cause death. Death usually occurs from cardiac arrhythmias, seizures, or severe hypotension.

J. **Mania:** Heterocyclic antidepressants can precipitate mania or rapid cycling in patients with bipolar disorder.

K. **Liver/Renal Disease:** Patients with hepatic or renal disease may require a lower dosage. Severe disease is a contraindication for TCAs.

L. **Discontinuation Syndrome:** Abrupt discontinuation of these agents may lead to transient dizziness, nausea, headache, diaphoresis, insomnia, and malaise. These effects are mostly related to cholinergic and serotonergic rebound. After prolonged treatment with heterocyclic agents, they should be tapered gradually over several weeks.

M. **Teratogenic Effects:** Heterocyclic antidepressants are classified as pregnancy class C. However, there is no evidence that TCAs cause major birth defects in humans. The impact of untreated depression on the mother and fetus must be considered when determining these risk benefit decisions. Lack of treatment during pregnancy can lead to severe adverse consequences for the woman and fetus. Data on behavioral teratogenicity is limited.

N. **Breast Feeding:** Heterocyclics are excreted in breast milk, and mothers should not breast feed when taking these agents.

V. **Drug Interactions**

A. **Plasma Level Increases:** Some of the new generation antidepressants, such as fluoxetine, can elevate heterocyclic antidepressants levels, leading to marked toxicity.

B. **Plasma Level Decreases:** Oral contraceptives, carbamazepine, barbiturates, chloral hydrate, and cigarette smoking can induce hepatic enzymes and lead to decreased levels of heterocyclics.

C. **Antihypertensives:** Heterocyclic agents can block the effects of antihypertensive agents, such as clonidine and propranolol.

D. **MAOIs:** The combination of heterocyclic agents with monoamine oxidase inhibitors can lead to a hypertensive crisis or a "serotonin syndrome," characterized by confusion, agitation, myoclonus, hyperreflexia, autonomic instability, delirium, coma, and even death. MAO inhibitors should be discontinued for 2 weeks before or after the use of a heterocyclic antidepressant.

E. **Anticholinergic Toxicity:** The combination of heterocyclics with other medications with anticholinergic properties can potentiate anticholinergic effects and may lead to delirium.

Amitriptyline (Elavil, Endep)

Indications: Depressive disorders, anxiety disorders, chronic pain, and insomnia.

Preparations: 10, 25, 50, 75, 100, 150 mg tablets; 10 mg/mL solution for IM injection.

Dosage:

Initial dosage: 25 mg qhs, then increase over 1-4 week period
Average dosage: 150-250 mg/day
Dosage range: 50-300 mg/day
Chronic Pain Syndromes: 25-300 mg qhs
Elderly: 25-200 mg/day

Half-life: 10-50 hr.

Therapeutic Level: 100-250 ng/mL (amitriptyline + nortriptyline)

Clinical Guidelines: Amitriptyline is widely used in the treatment of chronic pain and is effective in the prophylaxis of migraine headaches. Strong anticholinergic effects are often difficult for patients to tolerate. It is useful for insomnia, at a dosage of 25-100 mg qhs.

Clomipramine (Anafranil)

Indications: Depressive disorders and obsessive-compulsive disorder.
Preparations: 25, 50, 75 mg capsules.
Dosage:
- **Initial dosage:** 25 mg qhs, then increase over 1-4 week period.
- **Average dose:** 150-250 mg/day
- **Dosage Range:** 50-250 mg/day
- **Panic disorder:** 25-150 mg qhs

Half-life: 20-50 hr.
Therapeutic Level: 150-300 ng/mL
Clinical Guidelines: FDA approved for the treatment of OCD. OCD symptoms may require a longer duration of treatment (2-3 months) to achieve efficacy. Clomipramine may be especially useful in depressed patients with strong obsessional features. The side-effect profile (sedation and anticholinergic effects) often prevents patients from achieving an adequate dosage. Clomipramine has a higher risk of seizures than other TCAs.

Doxepin (Adapin, Sinequan)

Indications: Depressive disorders, anxiety disorders, insomnia, and chronic pain.
Preparations: 15, 25, 50, 75, 100, 150 mg tablets; 10 mg/mL liquid concentrate.
Dosage:
- **Initial dosage:** 25 mg qhs or bid, then increase over 1-4 week period
- **Average dosage:** 150-250 mg/day
- **Dosage range:** 25-300 mg/day
- **Elderly:** 15-200 mg/day
- **Insomnia:** 25-150 mg Qhs

Half-Life: 8-24 hr.
Therapeutic Levels: 100-250 ng/mL
Clinical Guidelines: Doxepin may be used in the treatment of chronic pain. It is one of the most sedating TCAs. The strong antihistamine properties of doxepin make it one of the most effective antipruritic agents available. It is useful for insomnia at a dosage of 25-150 mg qhs.

Imipramine (Tofranil)

Indications: Depressive disorders, anxiety disorders, enuresis, chronic pain.
Preparations: 10, 25, 50 mg tablets; 75, 100, 125, 150 mg capsules; 25 mg/2 mL solution for IM injection.
Dosage:
- **Initial dosage:** 25 mg qhs, then increase over 1-4 week period
- **Average dosage:** 150-250 mg/day
- **Dosage range:** 50-300 mg/day
- **Elderly:** 25-75 mg qhs (max 200 mg/day)

Half-Life: 5-25 hr.
Therapeutic Levels: 150-300 ng/mL (imipramine and desipramine)
Clinical Guidelines: Imipramine has well-documented effectiveness in the treatment of panic disorder. Imipramine is effective in the treatment of enuresis in children. The dosage for enuresis is usually 50-100 mg per day.

Trimipramine (Surmontil)

Indications: Depressive disorders, anxiety disorders.
Preparations: 25, 50, 100 mg capsules
Dosage:
- **Initial dosage:** 25 mg qhs, then increase over 1-4 week period.
- **Average dosage:** 150-200 mg/day
- **Dosage Range:** 50-300 mg/day
- **Elderly:** 25-50 mg qhs (max 200 mg/day)

Therapeutic Levels: Unknown
Clinical Guidelines: Trimipramine has no significant advantages over other TCAs.

References, see page 102.

Secondary Amine Tricyclic Antidepressants

Desipramine (Norpramin)

Indications: Depressive disorders, anxiety disorders, and chronic pain.
Preparations: 10, 25, 50, 75, 100, 150 mg tablets; 25, 50 mg capsules.
Dosage:
- **Initial dosage:** 25 mg qhs, then increase over 1-4 week period
- **Average dosage:** 150-250 mg/day
- **Dosage range:** 50-300 mg/day
- **Elderly:** 25-100 mg/day (max 200 mg/day)

Half-Life: 12-24 hr.
Therapeutic Levels: 125-300 ng/mL
Clinical Guidelines: Desipramine is one of the least sedating and least anticholinergic TCAs. It should be considered a first-line heterocyclic agents in elderly patients. Some patients may require AM dosing due to mild CNS activation.

Nortriptyline (Pamelor, Aventyl)

Indications: Depressive disorders, anxiety disorders, and chronic pain.
Preparations: 10, 25, 50, 75 mg capsules; 10 mg/5 m liquid concentrate.
Dosage:
- **Initial dosage:** 25 mg qhs, then increase over 1-4 week period
- **Average dosage:** 75-150 mg/day
- **Dosage range:** 25-150 mg/day
- **Elderly:** 10-75 mg/day (max 150 mg/day)

Half-Life: 18-44 hr.
Therapeutic Levels: 50-150 ng/mL
Clinical Guidelines: Nortriptyline is widely used in the treatment of chronic pain. It is one of the least likely TCAs to cause orthostatic hypotension and it is a good choice for elderly patients who require a TCA. Nortriptyline is the only antidepressant with known therapeutic serum levels. Patients generally respond at serum levels between 50-150 ng/mL.

Protriptyline (Vivactil)

Indications: Depressive disorders.
Preparations: 5, 10 mg tablets.
Dosage:
- **Initial dosage:** 5 mg qAM, then increase over several days to weeks.
- **Average dosage:** 15-40 mg/day

Dosage range: 10-60 mg/day
Elderly: 5 mg tid (max 40 mg/day)
Half-Life: 50-200 hr.
Therapeutic Levels: 75-200 ng/mL
Clinical Guidelines: Protriptyline is the least sedating and most activating TCA. Avoid giving near bedtime because it can cause insomnia. It has no advantage over other TCAs and is not commonly used.

References, see page 102.

Tetracyclic Antidepressants

Amoxapine (Asendin)

Indications: Depressive disorders, especially major depression with psychotic features.
Preparations: 25, 50, 100, 150 mg tablets.
Dosage:
 Initial dosage: 25-50 mg qhs, then increase gradually over 1-4 week period.
 Average dosage: 200-250 mg/day.
 Dosage range: 50-300 mg/day.
 Elderly: Start with 25 mg qhs; increase to 50 mg bid-tid (maximum 300 mg/day).
Half-Life: 8 hr.
Therapeutic Levels: 100-250 ng/mL
Clinical Guidelines: Amoxapine is related to the antipsychotic loxapine. Blockade of dopamine receptors may produce extrapyramidal symptoms (EPS) due to dopamine antagonism of its metabolite loxapine (eg, dystonia, akathisia, Parkinsonian symptoms). Dopamine receptor blockade can lead to hyper-prolactinemia with subsequent gynecomastia, galactorrhea, or amenorrhea. Amoxapine is associated with higher rates of seizure, arrhythmia, and fatality in overdose than many other antidepressants. The antipsychotic properties of loxapine may be useful in the treatment of major depression with psychotic features. It has added risks of dopamine antagonist side effects such as tardive dyskinesia.

Maprotiline (Ludiomil)

Indications: Depressive disorders.
Preparations: 25, 50, 75 mg tablets.
Dosage:
 Initial dosage: 75 mg qhs for 2 weeks, then increase in 25 mg increments over the next few weeks.
 Average dosage: 100-150 mg/day .
 Dosage range: 50-200 mg/day.
 Elderly: Start with 25 mg qhs. Increase to 50-75 qhs (max 100 mg/day).
Half-Life: 21-25 hr.
Therapeutic Levels: 150-300 ng/mL
Clinical Guidelines: Maprotiline is associated with higher rates of seizure, arrhythmia, and fatality in overdose than many other antidepressants. Avoid medications that lower seizure threshold, and avoid use in patients with risk of alcohol or sedative/hypnotic withdrawal syndrome. Do not use in patients with a history of seizures. The long half-life may necessitate a longer period of observation after overdose. Maprotiline is rarely used.

Mirtazapine (Remeron)

Indications: Depressive disorders.
Mechanism: Selective alpha-2 adrenergic antagonist that enhances noradrenergic and serotonergic neurotransmission.
Preparations: 15 and 30 mg scored tablets.
Soltabs: Orally disintegrating tablets (15, 30 and 45 mg).
Dosage:
Initial Dosage: Begin with 15 mg qhs and increase to 30 mg after several days to a maximum of 45 mg qhs.
Elderly: Begin with 7.5 mg qhs and increase by 7.5 mg each week to an average of 30 mg qhs.
Half-life: 20-40 hr.
Therapeutic levels: Not established.
Clinical Guidelines: Mirtazapine has little effect on sexual function. It may have some efficacy in anxiety disorders, and its antagonism of 5-HT3 receptors may help in patients with stomach upset. It has little effect on drugs metabolized by cytochrome P450 enzymes. Sedation is the most common side effect and may be marked initially, but usually decreases over the first week of treatment. Increase in appetite is frequent with an average weight gain of 2.0 kg after six weeks of treatment. Dry mouth, constipation, fatigue, dizziness, and orthostatic hypertension may occur. Agranulocytosis has occurred in two patients, and neutropenia has occurred in one patient during clinical trials with 2,800 patients. If a patient develops signs of an infection along with a low WBC, mirtazapine should be discontinued.
Drug Interactions: Mirtazapine has a low liability for drug interactions.

References, see page 102.

Monoamine Oxidase Inhibitors

I. Indications

A. Monoamine oxidase inhibitors(MAOIs) are used in the treatment of depressive and anxiety disorders. MAOIs are particularly useful in the treatment of major depression with atypical features, such as mood reactivity, increased appetite, hypersomnia, and sensitivity to interpersonal rejection.

B. These agents also have significant efficacy in anxiety disorders such as social phobia and panic disorder with agoraphobia and obsessive-compulsive disorder.

C. Given the dietary restrictions and risk of hypertensive crisis, most clinicians use MAOIs only after more conventional treatments have failed.

II. Pharmacology

A. Monoamine oxidase inhibitors irreversibly inhibit the enzyme, monoamine oxidase, located in the central nervous system, gut and platelets, leading to lack of degradation of monoamines.

B. The human body requires two weeks after discontinuing an MAOI to replenish the body with normal amounts of the monoamine oxidase enzyme.

C. MAOIs inhibit monamine oxidase in the gut wall which leads to increased absorption of tyramine. Tyramine can act as a false neurotransmitter and elevate blood pressure.

III. Clinical Guidelines

A. **Dietary Restrictions:** These agents require patients to adhere to a low tyramine diet in order to avoid a hypertensive crisis.

B. **Dose Titration:** In order to minimize side effects, these agents must be started at a low dose and titrated upward over days to weeks. This is a major disadvantage compared to SSRIs.

C. **Response Time:** These agents require at least 3-4 weeks for an adequate therapeutic trial and patients may respond after 6-8 weeks.

D. **Efficacy:** May be slightly more effective than other antidepressant treatments, especially with atypical depression.

E. **Clinical Utility:** Given the side-effect profile and dietary restrictions, these agents are generally reserved for use in patients who are refractory to other antidepressant treatments.

IV. Adverse Drug Reactions

A. **Alpha-1 Blockade:** Alpha-1 adrenergic blockade can lead to marked orthostatic hypotension. This is actually the most common side effect despite the fact that more clinical attention is focused on hypertensive crisis. This can be treated with salt supplements, support hose, or the mineralocorticoid, fludrocortisone. Dizziness and reflex tachycardia may also occur.

B. **Histaminic Blockade:** Antihistaminic properties can lead to sedation and significant weight gain.

C. **Hypertensive Crisis:** Hypertensive crisis from consuming tyramine containing foods is characterized by markedly elevated blood pressure, headache, sweating, nausea and vomiting, photophobia, autonomic instability, chest pain, cardiac arrhythmias, and even coma and death.

D. **Treatment of Hypertensive Crisis:** Treatment involves the use of nifedipine, 10 mg sublingual, while carefully monitoring blood pressure to make sure it does not drop too far. Alternatively, chlorpromazine, 50 mg orally, may be given. These agents can be given to patients to keep with them if they develop symptoms; however, they must be careful not to take these agents when they may be experiencing symptoms of hypotension. If patients present to the emergency room, they can be given phentolamine, 5 mg IV, followed by 0.25-0.5 mg IM every 4 to six hours as indicated.

E. **MAOI Diet:** Foods to be avoided: Soy sauce, sauerkraut, aged chicken or beef liver, aged cheese, fava beans, air-dried sausage or other meats, pickled or cured meat or fish, overripe fruit, canned figs, raisins, avocados, yogurt, sour cream, meat tenderizer, yeast extracts, caviar, and shrimp paste. Beer and wine are generally contraindicated; however, recent studies indicate that they contain very little tyramine.

F. **Pyridoxine Deficiency:** Pyridoxine deficiency, manifesting with paraesthesias, may occur and can be treated with vitamin B6, 50 mg per day.

G. **Overdose:** Overdose can be fatal and acidification of the urine or dialysis may be helpful along with other supportive treatment. Death may occur from arrhythmias, seizures or renal failure.

H. **Surgery:** Discontinue MAOIs 14 days before surgery to prevent hypertensive crisis from anesthetics.

I. **Mania:** MAOIs can induce mania or rapid cycling in patients with bipolar disorder.

J. **Comorbid Medical Illness:** Use with caution in patients with liver disease, abnormal liver function tests, cardiovascular disease, migraine headaches, renal disease, hyperthyroidism, or Parkinson's disease.

K. **Pregnancy:** Avoid use of MAOIs in pregnancy secondary to teratogenic potential.

L. **Miscellaneous:** Other side effects include, liver toxicity, agitation, dry mouth, constipation, seizures, sexual dysfunction, insomnia, and edema.

V. Drug Interactions

A. **Serotonergic Syndrome:** A serotonergic syndrome characterized by nausea, confusion, hyperthermia, autonomic instability, tremor, myoclonus, rigidity, seizures, coma and death, can occur when MAOIs are combined with SSRIs, TCAs, or carbamazepine. Wait fourteen days after discontinuing a MAOI before starting a TCA or SSRI. Discontinue sertraline, fluvoxamine and paroxetine for 14 days before beginning an MAOI and wait 5-6 weeks after discontinuing fluoxetine due to the long half-life of norfluoxetine.

B. **Opioids:** Opiate analgesics, especially meperidine, may lead to autonomic instability, delirium and death.

C. **Sympathomimetics:** Sympathomimetic agents such as amphetamines, cocaine, ephedrine, epinephrine, norepinephrine, dopamine, isoproterenol, methylphenidate, oxymetazoline, phenylephrine, phenylpropanolamine metaraminol can lead to a hypertensive crisis.

D. **Antihypertensives:** Antihypertensive agents can further increase the likelihood of hypotension.

E. **Oral Hypoglycemics:** MAOIs can potentiate decreases in blood glucose when combined with oral hypoglycemics.

Phenelzine (Nardil)

Indications: Effective for atypical depression. Also used for anxiety disorders such as panic disorder with agoraphobia, social phobia, and obsessive-compulsive disorder.
Preparations: 15 mg tablets.
Dosage:
Initial dosage: 15 mg bid; increase by 15 mg/day each week.
Average dosage: 30-60 mg/day.
Dosage range: 15-90 mg/day.
Elderly: Start with 7.5-15 mg/day; max 60 mg/day.
Therapeutic Levels: Not established.
Clinical Guidelines: Major morbidity and mortality risks are associated with MAOI use. Phenelzine is associated with a higher incidence of weight gain, drowsiness, dry mouth, and sexual dysfunction than tranylcypromine.

Tranylcypromine (Parnate)

Indications: Approved for atypical depression. Also used for anxiety disorders, such as panic disorder with agoraphobia, social phobia, and obsessive-compulsive disorder.
Preparations: 10 mg tablets
Dosage:
Initial dosage: 10 mg bid. Increase by 10 mg/day each week.
Average dosage: 20-40 mg/day.
Dosage range: 10-60 mg/day.
Elderly: Start with 5-10 mg/day; max 30-40 mg/day.
Therapeutic Levels: Not established.
Clinical Guidelines: Major morbidity and mortality risks are associated with MAO-I use. Phenelzine is associated with higher incidences of weight gain, drowsiness, dry mouth, and sexual dysfunction than tranylcypromine. Tranylcypromine is more likely to cause insomnia than phenelzine.

References, see page 102.

Antipsychotics

Clinical Use of Antipsychotics

I. **Indications:** Antipsychotic agents (also referred to as neuroleptics) are indicated for the treatment of schizophrenia. Antipsychotics are also used for schizoaffective disorder, mood disorders with psychotic symptoms, and brief psychotic disorder. They often improve functioning in patients with dementia or delirium when psychotic symptoms are present. They are also frequently used for treatment of substance induced psychotic disorders and in psychotic symptoms associated with certain personality disorders (borderline).

II. **Pharmacology:** Typical and atypical antipsychotics are distinguished by their unique receptor binding profiles primarily with dopamine and serotonin receptors. Typical antipsychotic agents have been the first-line treatment for schizophrenia. New atypical antipsychotics, however, are challenging this first-line position because of their greater tolerability and increased efficacy.

- **A.** The efficacy of typical antipsychotic agents is primarily related to their binding to dopamine D2 receptors.
  - **1.** Typical antipsychotic agents may be divided into high-, moderate-, and low-potency categories based on their level of dopamine receptor antagonism.
  - **2.** All agents within the typical antipsychotic category are equally effective.
    - **a.** High-potency agents have the highest affinity for D2 receptors and are effective at relatively lower doses.
    - **b.** Low-potency agents have lower D2 affinity and require larger doses to elicit an antipsychotic effect.
- **B.** Atypical agents (serotonin-dopamine antagonists, SDAs) are distinguished by their prominent antagonism at the serotonin 2A receptor in addition to D2 blockade. The ratio of serotonin to dopamine blockade is generally high for these agents. These agents are also unique in that there appears to be more selectivity for the mesolimbic dopamine pathway, which is thought to be a site of antipsychotic action. There is relatively less action on the nigrostriatal pathway where extrapyramidal side effects are thought to originate. As a group these drugs have a therapeutic dose range that allows for the antipsychotic effect without inducing significant extrapyramidal symptoms.
  - **1.** Clozapine is an antagonist of serotonin-2A, alpha-1, dopamine-1, 2, and 4 receptors. Clozapine also possesses significant antihistamine and anticholinergic properties, leading to a side-effect profile similar to that of the typical low-potency agents.
  - **2.** SDAs include risperidone (Risperdal), olanzapine (Zyprexa), ziprasidone (Geodon) and quetiapine (Seroquel).
- **C. Pharmacokinetics**
  - **1.** After oral absorption, peak plasma levels of antipsychotics usually occur within 2-4 hours. Liquid preparations are absorbed more quickly. IM injections reach peak levels in 30-60 minutes.
  - **2.** Antipsychotic agents undergo extensive hepatic metabolism. Typically 50% of the antipsychotic is excreted via enterohepatic circulation and

50% through the kidneys.

3. Antipsychotics are 85-90% protein bound and highly lipophilic.
4. Half-lives generally range from 5-50 hours. Steady state plasma levels are established in 4-10 days.

III. Clinical Guidelines

A. Choosing an Antipsychotic Agent

1. In general, the choice of neuroleptic should be made based on past history of response to a neuroleptic and side effects.
2. Atypical antipsychotics have gained acceptance as first-line drugs for treatment of psychosis. They can contribute to superior long-term outcome in treatment of schizophrenia compared to typicals. At least two weeks of treatment is required before a significant antipsychotic effect is achieved.
3. Poor response of negative symptoms (affective flattening) is an indication for a trial of an atypical agent. Negative symptoms can occur secondary to treatment with typical neuroleptics.
4. Patients with tardive dyskinesia (TD) should be considered for treatment with an atypical agent to avoid progression of neurological impairment.
   a. Clozapine is not associated with TD.
   b. Olanzapine (Zyprexa), risperidone (Risperdal), quetiapine (Seroquel) and ziprasidone (Geodon) have significantly reduced incidences of TD.

B. Efficacy

1. **Positive Symptoms:** With the exception of clozapine, no differences have been clearly shown in the efficacy of typical and atypical agents in the treatment of positive symptoms (eg, hallucinations, delusions, disorganization)
2. **Negative Symptoms:** Atypical agents may be more effective in the treatment of negative symptoms (eg, affective flattening, anhedonia, avolition) associated with psychotic disorders. The evidence, however, does not conclusively support this view.
3. **Treatment-Resistant Psychosis:** Patients failing to respond to adequate trials of typical agents may respond to an atypical agent. Thirty percent of poor responders to typical agents show significant improvement when treated with clozapine.

IV. Adverse Drug Reactions

A. **Tardive dyskinesia (TD)** is a long-term, often permanent, neurological impairment resulting from extensive use of typical antipsychotics. Atypical agents, however, have minimal risk of TD.

B. **Neuroleptic malignant syndrome** is an uncommon, yet potentially fatal, adverse reaction to typical antipsychotics. Although some risk of neuroleptic malignant syndrome may be present with risperidone use, this risk is minimal with clozapine.

C. Side Effects

1. The older typical antipsychotics have traditionally been classified according to their potency. Chlorpromazine is an example of low-potency drug where a dose fo 500-1000 mg is often used while haloperidol is an example of high-potency antipsychotic (5-10 mg is a usual dose). Low-potency typical antipsychotic agents and clozapine have more troublesome side effects than high-potency agents because

of greater antagonism of cholinergic, adrenergic, and histaminergic receptors. High-potency typical agents, however, have more frequent extrapyramidal side effects because of potent antagonism of dopamine receptors. The atypical agents generally have much lower antagonism of cholinergic, adrenergic and histaminergic receptors. Side-effect profiles resulting from antagonism of these receptor pathways is summarized as follows:

a. **Muscarinic (cholinergic):** Dry mouth, constipation, urinary retention, blurred vision, precipitation of narrow angle glaucoma, ECG changes
b. **Alpha-1 Adrenergic:** Orthostatic hypotension, lightheadedness, tachycardia, sedation and sexual dysfunction.
c. **Histamine-1:** Sedation, weight gain, fatigue.
d. **Dopamine-2:** Extrapyramidal Parkinsonian symptoms (eg, dystonic reactions, masked facies, tremor, shuffling gait); hyperprolactinemia (not with clozapine), dystonic reaction, akathisia (restlessness).
e. **Serotonin-1C:** May mediate weight gain for some atypical agents (olanzapine).
f. **Non-specific Side Effects:** Include hyperthermia, hypothermia, hepatitis, jaundice, photosensitivity, lowered seizure threshold, hematologic changes, hepatitis, and rash.

D. Management of Side Effects

1. Neuroleptic Malignant Syndrome (NMS) is an uncommon side effect with possible fatal outcome. NMS is marked by elevated temperature, autonomic instability, delirium, and rigid muscle tone, developing over 24-72 hours. Risk factors for neuroleptic malignant syndrome include dehydration, heat exhaustion, and poor nutrition.
2. **Agranulocytosis.** Most common with clozapine (1-2% incidence). Clozapine should be discontinued if WBC drops below 3,000/mcL or 50% of the patient's normal level, or if the absolute granulocyte count drops below 1,500/mcL.
3. **Tardive Dyskinesia (TD)** is a neurological impairment, primarily limited to patients with a history of chronic neuroleptic administration (greater than two months). TDs are characterized by involuntary dyskinetic movements that may affect any striate muscle and may result in permanent dysfunction of facial (eg, lingual, perioral), truncal, esophageal, neck, or extremity motor function. Risk for TD increases by 1% with each year of antipsychotic treatment. Treatment may include the following:
   a. Quantify the degree of neurological dysfunction by using a rating scale, such as the abnormal involuntary movement scale (AIMS).
   b. Reduce or stop antipsychotic if possible.
   c. If continued antipsychotic is necessary, consider change to an atypical agent.
   d. Some studies suggest that vitamin E offers modest benefits in prevention and treatment of TD, particularly if initiated early.
4. Dystonic reactions are characterized by painful, acute involuntary muscle spasms. They are common side effects of typical antipsychotic agents. Dystonic reactions commonly involve the extremities, neck (torticollis), and ocular muscles (oculogyric crisis). The muscle contractions are not life threatening unless they involve airway

passages (eg, larynx) and lead to airway obstruction. Treatment may include:

a. **Intramuscular or Intravenous Antiparkinsonian Agent**
   (1) Benztropine (Cogentin), 1-2 mg PO, IM, IV **or**
   (2) Diphenhydramine (Benadryl), 50 mg PO, IM, IV.

b. Consider change of antipsychotic to relieve patient fears. Prophylaxis against further episodes of dystonia is accomplished with an oral anticholinergic agent such as benztropine (Cogentin), 2 mg PO bid for one to two months.

5. If dystonic reactions occur after discontinuing anticholinergic agent, longer prophylactic treatment should be provided (eg, 3-6 months).
6. Drug-induced parkinsonian symptoms include bradykinesia, tremor, cogwheel rigidity, masked facies, and festinating gait. Treatments include:
   a. Decreasing antipsychotic dose.
   b. Use of anticholinergic drug (eg, benztropine).
   c. Changing to lower-potency or atypical agent.
   d. Tremor can be treated with propranolol, 10-40 mg PO bid to qid.
7. Akathisia is characterized by an intense sense of restlessness or anxiety. Treatments include:
   a. Decreasing antipsychotic dose.
   b. Trial of anticholinergic agent (eg, benztropine 2 mg PO bid).
   c. Trial of beta-adrenergic antagonist such as propranolol, 10-40 mg PO bid to qid.
   d. Trial of a benzodiazepine such as clonazepam, 0.5 mg PO bid.
   e. Consider changing to lower-potency or atypical agent.

E. **Overdose**

1. Death is uncommon with antipsychotic overdose. Risk of fatality is increased with concurrent use of alcohol or other CNS depressants.
2. Mesoridazine, pimozide and thioridazine are associated with a greatest risk of fatality because of heart block and ventricular tachycardia.
3. CNS depression, hypotension, seizures, fever, ECG changes, hypothermia, and hyperthermia are possible.
4. Treatment may include gastric lavage, catharsis, IV diazepam for treatment of seizure, and medical treatment of hypotension.

F. **Drug Interactions**

1. **Antacids and cimetidine.** Absorption of antipsychotics may be inhibited.
2. **Anticholinergics, antihistamines, antiadrenergics.** Additive effects.
3. **Antihypertensives** may potentiate hypotension (eg, ACE Inhibitors and alpha-methyldopa); may inhibit neuronal uptake of clonidine and alpha-methyldopa.
4. **Anticonvulsants** may induce metabolism and decrease level of antipsychotic; phenothiazines may decrease metabolism/ increase level of phenytoin.
5. **Antidepressants** tricyclics and SSRIs may reduce metabolism and increase levels of antipsychotics.
6. **Antipsychotics** may increase levels of tricyclics.
7. **Barbiturates** by enzyme induction levels of antipsychotics may be reduced; may cause respiratory depression.
8. **Beta-blockers.** Propranolol increases blood levels of antipsychotics.

9. **Bromocriptine** may worsen psychotic symptoms. Antipsychotics will decrease effect of bromocriptine.
10. **Cigarettes** may increase metabolism and decrease level of antipsychotics.
11. **CNS depressants** (including benzodiazepines, narcotics, and alcohol) enhance sedative effects of antipsychotics.
12. **Digoxin** absorption may be increased.
13. **Isoniazid** may increase risk of hepatic toxicity.
14. **L-Dopa.** Effects blocked by dopamine antagonists.
15. **Lithium.** Possible risk of neuroleptic-induced encephalopathic syndrome or neurotoxicity.
16. **MAO inhibitors** will potentiate hypotensive effects of antipsychotics.
17. **Metrizamide** decreases seizure threshold. Avoid concomitant use with typical agents.
18. **Oral Contraceptives** may increase levels of antipsychotics.
19. **Stimulants.** Amphetamine may worsen psychotic symptoms. Antipsychotics will lessen effects of stimulants.
20. **Warfarin.** Highly protein-bound, may alter antipsychotic levels; levels may be decreased leading to decreased bleeding time.

G. Preexisting Medical Conditions:

1. **Cardiac History.** Use high-potency agent (other than pimozide) or atypicals (other than clozapine) to avoid conduction abnormalities.
2. **Elderly** patients are more sensitive to side effects; atypical drugs should be utilized initially. Most experience is with risperidone, which can be used in low doses (0.5 mg). If typical agents are to be used, start with a low dose of a high-potency agent (0.5 mg of haloperidol) and increase slowly.
3. **Hematologic Disorder.** Clozapine is contraindicated.
4. **Hepatic, Renal, Cardiac, Respiratory Disease.** Use antipsychotics with caution; monitor renal, cardiac, and liver function.
5. **Parkinson's Disease.** Atypical agents are preferred due to selectivity for mesolimbic dopamine tract.
6. **Prostatic Hypertrophy.** Agents with high anticholinergic activity are contraindicated.
7. **Seizure History.** Some studies suggest that molindone may have lower seizure risk more than other antipsychotics. Atypicals are also indicated for patients with a seizure disorder. Avoid loxapine and clozapine.
8. **Pregnancy.** Phenothiazines may increase risk of anomalies. Avoid low-potency agents. Fluphenazine, haloperidol, trifluoperazine, and perphenazine are associated with lower risks during pregnancy.

References, see page 102.

Atypical Antipsychotics

I. **Indications**

A. Atypical antipsychotics are indicated for psychotic disorders including schizophrenia, schizoaffective disorder, brief psychotic disorders, and psychotic symptoms associated with mood disorders, substance abuse, organic brain syndromes, dementia, and personality disorders.

B. Clozapine has been demonstrated to be more effective for positive symptoms in treatment-resistant psychotic patients.

II. **Pharmacology**

A. The primary distinguishing property of the currently available atypical agents (serotonin-dopamine antagonists, SDAs) is prominent antagonism at the serotonin 2A receptor in addition to D2 blockade.

B. The ratio of serotonin to dopamine blockade is generally high for these agents. These agents are also unique in that there appears to be more selectivity for the mesolimbic dopamine pathway, which is thought to be important in mediating antipsychotic action.

C. There is relatively less action on the nigrostriatal pathway where extrapyramidal side effects are thought to originate. As a group these drugs have a therapeutic dose range that allows for the antipsychotic effect without inducing significant extrapyramidal symptoms.

D. Clozapine is an antagonist of serotonin-2A, alpha-1, and dopamine-1, 2, and 4 receptors. Clozapine also possesses significant antihistamine and anticholinergic properties, resulting in a side-effect profile that is similar to that of the typical low-potency agents.

E. Aripiprazole (Abilify), risperidone (Risperdal), olanzapine (Zyprexa), ziprasidone (Geodon) and quetiapine (Seroquel) are available SDAs.

III. **Clinical Guidelines**

A. Although atypical agents have been reserved for patients who have failed treatment with one typical agent, clozapine should be reserved for patients who have failed to respond to two different antipsychotics. Atypical antipsychotics have gained acceptance as first-line drugs for treatment of psychosis. These agents produce superior long-term outcomes compared to typicals in the treatment of schizophrenia.

B. Atypical agents are clearly indicated if a patient develops significant side effects when treated with typical agents.

C. Poor response of negative symptoms of psychosis is an indication for a trial of an atypical agent. Some negative symptoms can be secondary to treatment with typical neuroleptics. For example, neuroleptic induced Parkinsonism being misinterpreted as flat affect. Although not firmly established, the atypical agents may be efficacious for primary negative symptoms.

D. Patients with tardive dyskinesia (TD) should be considered for treatment with an atypical agent to avoid progression of neurological impairment.

1. Clozapine is not associated with TDs.
2. Aripiprazole (Abilify), olanzapine (Zyprexa), risperidone (Risperdal), quetiapine (Seroquel) and ziprasidone (Geodon) have a significantly reduced incidence of TD.

IV. **Treatment**

A. Initial treatment should be continued for four to six weeks. If there is no response after this period, a change to an alternate medication is warranted.

B. **Medically compromised patients**. Atypical agents are indicated in patients with conditions that predispose them to increased sensitivity to side effects of typical agents (eg, dementia, diabetes).

V. **Adverse Drug Reactions**

A. With the exception of clozapine the atypical agents are very well tolerated. There is a much lower occurrence of extrapyramidal symptoms.

B. The atypical agents are expected to have a very low incidence of neuroleptic malignant syndrome and tardive dyskinesia.

Aripiprazole (Abilify)

Class: Quinolinone

Mechanism: Aripiprazole is a new partial agonist at the dopamine D_2 and the serotonin 5-HT_{1A} receptors, and it is an antagonist of the serotonin 5-HT_{2A} receptor.

Indications: Aripiprazole is indicated for psychotic disorders that are refractory to treatment with typical antipsychotics. They are indicated for patients with tardive dyskinesia or severe side effects associated with other neuroleptics.

Preparations: 10 mg, 15 mg, 20 mg, and 30 mg tablets; no IM preparation is available.

Dosage:

Initial Dosage: 10-15 mg qAM and increased to 20 to 30 mg per day after 2-4 weeks if needed; however, clinical trials have not found greater efficacy for doses above 10-15 mg.

Maintenance: 10-30 mg per day.

Elderly: While aripiprazole clearance is reduced by 20% in patients over 65, no dosage adjustment is required or recommended at this time. Begin with a lower dosage in debilitated elderly patients.

Metabolism: Half-life is 75 hours for aripiprazole and 94 hours for its active metabolite, dehydro-aripiprazole. Hepatic metabolism is mainly through CYP2D6 and CYP3A4. Poor metabolizers who lack CYP2D6, have an 80% increase in aripiprazole plasma levels and a 30% decrease in dehyro-aripiprazole levels compared to normal.

Therapeutic Level: Not established.

Side-Effect Profile: The most common side effect is nausea, with occasional vomiting, which usually resolves within one week. The incidence of sedation is low, but can occur especially at higher dosages. Anxiety and insomnia may occur, especially early in treatment. Orthostatic hypotension occurs rarely. The incidence of extrapyramidal symptoms is comparable to placebo. Aripiprazole does not appear to effect QT_C intervals.

Clinical Guidelines: Aripiprazole should be given in the morning due to lack of sedation compared to other agents. It is recommended that aripiprazole can be added to a current antipsychotic medication regimen with tapering of the other antipsychotic gradually over time. Early data seems to indicate a low liability for weight gain, or changes in glucose or lipid levels. Aripiprazole does not elevate serum prolactin.

Drug Interactions:

A. Coadminisration of aripiprazole with potent inhibitors of CYP2D6, such as quinidine, fluoxetine or paroxetine, can markedly increase blood levels (112% with quinidine) and requires dosage adjustment to one-half of its normal dosage.

B. Ketoconazole or other potent inhibitors of CYP3A4 require adjusting aripiprazole to one-half of its normal dosage.

C. Carbamazepine, a CYP 3A4 inducer, can lower plasma aripiprazole levels and the dose of aripiprazole should be doubled when coadministered.

D. Aripiprazole does not appear to effect levels of other cytochrome P450 substrates metabolized by CYP2D6,CYP2C9, CYP2C19, or CYP3A4.

Clozapine (Clozaril)

Class: Dibenzodiazepine

Mechanism: Multiple receptor antagonism: serotonin 5HT2A receptor, dopamine D1, D2, and D4 receptors.

Indications: Psychotic disorders which are refractory to treatment with typical antipsychotics. They are indicated for patients with tardive dyskinesia or severe side effects associated with other neuroleptics.

Preparations: 25, 100 mg scored tablets; no IM preparation available

Dosage:

Initial Dosage: 25 mg bid, then increase by 25-50 mg every 2-3 days to achieve total daily dose of between 300-600 mg. Dose may need to be given tid if side effects occur.

Maintenance: 400-600 mg/day; some patients may require higher doses but rarely more than 900 mg/day.

Metabolism: Half-life 11 hours, hepatic metabolism, CYP1A2.

Therapeutic Level: >350 ng/mL.

Side-Effect Profile: Orthostatic hypotension (high), sedation (high), anticholinergic (high), extrapyramidal symptoms (absent). Most common: sedation, dizziness, hypotension, tachycardia, constipation, hyperthermia, hypersalivation. Hypersalivation can be treated with anticholinergic agents.

Clinical Guidelines: Clozapine does not cause tardive dyskinesia or neuroleptic malignant syndrome. Clozapine is often effective against symptoms that are resistant to typical agents. It is more effective than typical agents in treatment of the negative symptoms of schizophrenia. Clozapine may decrease the risk of suicide in schizophrenia and an FDA advisory panel has recommended expanding the indications for clozapine to include suicide prevention.

Drug Interactions:

A. **Cimetidine (Tagamet)** may increase clozapine levels. Use ranitidine (Zantac) instead.

B. **Fluvoxamine** can double clozapine levels

C. TCAs can increase risk for seizures, cardiac changes, sedation

Contraindications: Clozapine is contraindicated in patients with granulocytopenia or a history of agranulocytosis induced by clozapine. Do not use clozapine with drugs that suppress bone marrow or have a risk of agranulocytosis (eg, carbamazepine, sulfonamides, captopril).

Adverse Effects:

- **A.** Clozapine has a 1-2% incidence of agranulocytosis. Patients should be instructed to report the onset of fever, sore throat, weakness or other signs of infection promptly. Discontinue the drug if the WBC drops below 3,000/mcL, or 50% of patient's normal count, or if granulocyte count drops below 1,500/mcL. Once the WBC normalizes, the patient may be rechallenged. WBC should be monitored weekly for the first 3 months of treatment. Thereafter, monitoring can be reduced to every 2 weeks.
- **B.** A 5% incidence of seizure has been noted in patients taking more than 600 mg/day of clozapine. If seizures develop, discontinue drug use and consider restarting with concurrent use of divalproex sodium (Depakote).
- **C.** Rare myocarditis(5-100 cases/100,000 patient years) has been seen especially during, but not limited to the first month of clozapine treatment. Consider myocarditis if patients present with unexplained fatigue, dyspnea, tachypnea, fever, chest pain, palpitations, other signs of heart failure, or ECG changes such as ST-T wave abnormalities or arrhythmias.
- **D.** Use clozapine with caution and at low doses in patients with hepatic or renal disease.
- **E.** Monitor patients for hypotension and tachycardia. When discontinuing clozapine, the dosage should be tapered over two weeks because anticholinergic rebound may occur.

Risperidone (Risperdal)

Class: Benzisoxazole.

Mechanism: Antagonist of serotonin-2A, dopamine-2 and alpha-1 receptors.

Preparations: 0.25, 0.5, 1, 2, 3, 4 mg tablets (1 mg tablet is scored); 1 mg/mL oral soln; the long-acting IM preparation (Consta) is likely to be approved in 2003.

Dosage:

Initial Dosage: 1 mg bid, then increase by 1 mg every 2-3 days to 2-3 mg bid.

Acute agitation: No acute IM dose available.

Maintenance: 2-8 mg bid, many patients can be treated with 4 mg given as a single dose.

Long-acting IM formulation (Consta)(FDA approval pending):
25 - 50 mg IM every month (no evidence to increase beyond 50 mg).

Elderly: reduced dosage (1-4 mg/day).

Metabolism: Half-life is 3-20 hours. Hepatic metabolism to an active metabolite. Renal clearance. No risperidone-specific drug interactions.

Therapeutic Level: Not established.

Side-Effect Profile: Orthostatic hypotension and reflex tachycardia (alpha 1 receptor mediated, minimized with slow upward titration), insomnia, and agitation are the most frequent. Incidence of extrapyramidal symptoms is very low. Risperidone can cause weight gain and increase prolactin levels (usually not clinically significant). May prolong QT interval.

Clinical Guidelines: Risperidone is generally very well tolerated. A low incidence of extrapyramidal symptoms is associated with doses less than 6 mg. Risperidone may be given in once-a-day dose schedules. There is increasing experience with successful use of risperidone in elderly populations. There have been a number of case reports of neuroleptic malignant syndrome.

Olanzapine (Zyprexa, Zydis)

Class: Thienobenzodiazepine
Mechanism: Antagonist of serotonin-2A, dopamine-1, 2, 3, 4, alpha-1, histamine-1, and muscarinic-1 receptors.
Preparations: Zyprexa: 2.5, 5, 7.5, 10, 15 mg tablets.
Zydis: 2.5, 5, 7.5 10, 15 mg orally disintegrating tablets.
IM Zyprexa (for acute use): FDA approval pending.
Dosage:
Initial dosage: 10 mg/day.
Range: 5-20 mg/day, although some patients may require higher doses.
IM: 5 -10 mg IM every 2 hours (maximum dose not determined).
Therapeutic Level: Not established.
Metabolism: Half-life is 21-50 hours. Hepatic metabolism (primarily through P450 1A2) to inactive metabolites. Olanzapine levels may be decreased by tobacco use and by carbamazepine (1A2 induction). Olanzapine levels may be increased by fluvoxamine (1A2 inhibition). Dose should be reduced in the elderly. Olanzapine levels tend to be higher in females.
Side-Effect Profile: Most common side effects are drowsiness, dry mouth, akathisia, and insomnia. Less frequent are orthostatic hypotension, light-headedness, nausea, and tremor. Weight gain is common with olanzapine. Increases in lipids and blood glucose are also observed. There are reports of new onset diabetes and diabetic ketoacidosis. Despite a similar chemical structure to clozapine, there is no evidence of hemotoxicity.
Clinical Guidelines: Very well tolerated. No titration is required and many patients can be treated with once a day dosing. Weight gain can occur. Because of pharmacokinetic variability, doses beyond 20 mg/day may be required in some patients.

Quetiapine (Seroquel)

Class: Dibenzothiazepine.
Mechanism: Quetiapine (Seroquel) is an antagonist at the serotonin-2A, dopamine-2, alpha-1 and 2, and histamine-1 receptors.
Preparations: 25 mg, 100 mg, and 200 mg tablets.
Dosage:
Initial dosage: 25-50 mg bid, increased by 25-50 mg every 1 to 3 days to a total daily dose of 400-600 mg.
Maintenance: Required daily dose can range between 150-750 mg.
Elderly: Clearance is reduced by 40% in elderly; dosage should be reduced in this population.
Therapeutic Level: Not established.
Metabolism: Half-life is 6 hours, hepatic metabolism (P450 3A4), no active

metabolites. Low potential for drug interactions.

Side-Effect Profile: Orthostatic hypotension may occur during initial dose titration due to alpha-blockade. Somnolence and weight gain may occur due to H_1 blockade. Dyspepsia, abdominal pain, and dry mouth may also occur. There are reports of new onset diabetes or diabetic ketoacidosis.

Clinical Guidelines: May be effective for primary negative symptoms of schizophrenia. Minimal weight gain. Well tolerated. No anticholinergic side effects. Very low incidence of EPS. No sustained elevation of prolactin. Requires bid or tid dosing.

Ziprasidone (Geodon)

Class: Benzisothiazolyl piperazine.

Indications: Psychotic disorders.

Mechanism: D2, D3, 5HT2A, 5HT1A antagonism; also blocks reuptake of monoamines.

Preparations: 40 mg capsules, IM formulation: 20 mg/ml dose vial.

Maintenance Dosage: Target dose is between 40-80 mg bid;

IM Preparation: 10 mg IM every 2 hours or 20 mg IM every 4 hours to maximum daily dose of 40 mg.

Therapeutic Level: Not established.

Metabolism: Inactive metabolites, half-life 4 hours. Low potential for drug interactions.

Side-Effect Profile: Dizziness, nausea, and postural hypotension are the most common side effects. Prolactin elevation can occur. Sedation is more common with the IM preparation.

Advantages/ Disadvantages: Very low incidence of extrapyramidal symptoms. Minimal incidence of cardiovascular problems. Prolactin elevation is minimal. The incidence of weight gain, lipid abnormalities, and glucose intolerance appears to be lower than other atypical antipsychotics. Ziprasidone can increase QT interval. While there are no reports linking this to cardiac arrhythmias, caution should be exercised in patients with pre-existing increased QT interval (from medications or cardiac disease). These patients should have a baseline ECG. QT prolongation has not been observed with the IM formulation.

References, see page 102.

High-Potency Antipsychotics

Side-Effect Profile: Orthostatic hypotension (low), sedation (low), anticholinergic (low). Extrapyramidal symptoms are frequent.
Clinical Guidelines: High-potency agents have less sedative, hypotensive, and anticholinergic side effects. Many patients require concurrent use of an antiparkinsonian agent (eg, benztropine) to control extrapyramidal symptoms.

Fluphenazine (Prolixin)

Class: Piperazine
Indications: Psychotic disorders.
Preparations: 1, 2.5, 5, 10 mg tablets; 2.5, 5 mg/mL oral solution; 2.5 mg/mL parenteral solution (IM); 25 mg/mL decanoate (IM).
Dosage:

- **Initial:** 2.5-10 mg/day, may be titrated to 40 mg/day.
- **Maintenance:** 10-20 mg/day.
- **Acute agitation:** 2.5-5 mg IM, should not exceed daily dose of 10 mg IM
- **Elderly:** 0.5-2mg bid/tid.
- **Chronic noncompliance**: Switch to decanoate formulation. Give 12.5 mg IM of decanoate every two weeks for every 10 mg of oral dose.

Potency: (equivalent to 100 mg chlorpromazine): 2 mg.
Metabolism: Hepatic metabolism, half-life 10-20 hours. The decanoate formulation has a typical duration of action of 2 weeks.
Therapeutic Level: Not established.
Clinical Guidelines: Fluphenazine is a weak antiemetic. Decanoate formulation available.

Haloperidol (Haldol)

Class: Butyrophenone
Indications: Psychotic disorders, Tourette's Syndrome.
Preparations:
Haloperidol tablets: 0.5, 1, 2, 5, 10, 20 mg.
Haloperidol lactate: 2 mg/mL conc. (PO), 5 mg/mL soln. (IM).
Haloperidol decanoate: 50, 100 mg/mL (IM - depot).
Dosage:

- **Initial:** 5-10 mg/day.
- **Maintenance:** 5-20 mg/day.
- **Acute agitation:** 5.0 - 10 mg IM. Should not exceed daily dose of 20 mg IM.
- **Elderly:** 0.5-2 mg bid/tid.
- **Chronic noncompliance:** Switch to haloperidol decanoate at 10-20 times the daily dose, given on monthly basis. Maximum initial dose of 100 mg/day IM. Give balance of dose 4-5 days later if necessary. Do not give more than

3 mL per injection site.

Tourette's disorder in children: 0.05- 0.1 mg/kg in 2 or 3 divided doses

Potency: (equivalent to 100 mg chlorpromazine): 2 mg

Metabolism: Hepatic metabolism to active metabolite. Half-life 10–20 hours. Duration of action of decanoate is approximately 4 weeks.

Therapeutic Level: 5-20 ng/mL..

Major Safety Concerns: High incidence of extrapyramidal symptoms. May possibly lower seizure threshold in patients with a history of seizures.

Pimozide (Orap)

Class: Diphenylbutylpiperdines.

Indications: Psychotic disorders, Tourette's Syndrome.

Preparations: 2.0 mg tablets.

Dosage:

Tourette's: 0.5-1 mg bid, then increase dose every other day as needed (max 0.2 mg/kg/day or 10 mg).

Antipsychotic maintenance: 1-10 mg/day.

Potency: (equivalent to 100 mg chlorpromazine): 1 mg.

Metabolism: Hepatic metabolism. Half-life 55 hours.

Therapeutic Level: Not established.

Contraindications: Pimozide is contraindicated in patients with a history of cardiac arrhythmia or with drugs that prolong QT interval.

Major Safety Concerns: Pimozide may cause ECG changes, including prolongation of QT interval, T-wave inversion, and appearance of U waves and alter effects of antiarrhythmic agents.

Cardiac side effects of pimozide make haloperidol safer first-line treatment for Tourette's Syndrome. Use caution in patients with a history of hypokalemia.

Thiothixene (Navane)

Class: Thioxanthene.

Indications: Psychotic disorders.

Preparations: Capsules: 1, 2, 5, 10, 20 mg.

Thiothixene hydrochloride: 5 mg/mL oral solution; 5 mg/mL parenteral (IM).

Dosage:

Initial dosage: 2-5 mg bid-tid. Titrate to 20-40 mg/day (max 60 mg/day).

Maintenance: 5-20 mg/day.

Acute agitation: 5 mg IM 4 hour prn.

Elderly: 1-15 mg/day.

Potency (equivalent to 100 mg chlorpromazine): 5 mg.

Metabolism: Hepatic metabolism. Half-life 10 – 20 hours.

Therapeutic Level: Not established. Some suggest 2-57 ng/mL.

Major Safety Concerns: May produce ocular pigmentary changes. Periodic ophthalmological examination is recommended.

Trifluoperazine (Stelazine)

Class: Piperazine.
Preparations: 1, 2, 5, 10 mg tablets; 10 mg/mL oral solution, 2 mg/mL soln. (IM).
Dosage:

- **Initial:** 2-5 mg bid-tid. Titrate to 20-40 mg/day (max 60 mg/day).
- **Maintenance:** 5-20 mg/day.
- **Acute agitation:** 5 mg IM q 4 hour prn (max of 20 mg/day). Do not repeat dosage in less than 4 hrs.
- **Elderly:** 1-15 mg/day.

Potency (equivalent to 100 mg chlorpromazine): 5 mg.
Metabolism: Hepatic metabolism. Half-life 10–20 hours.
Therapeutic Level: Not established.
Clinical Guidelines: Associated with few ECG changes.

References, see page 102.

Mid-Potency Antipsychotics

Side-Effect Profile: Orthostatic hypotension (moderate), sedation (moderate), anticholinergic (moderate), extrapyramidal symptoms (high). Anticholinergic side effects of mid-potency agents lessen the need for medication to control extrapyramidal side effects. Neuroleptic malignant syndrome, tardive dyskinesia, and dystonic reactions are possible.

Loxapine (Loxitane)

Class: Dibenzoxapine.
Preparations: 5, 10, 25, 50 mg capsules; 25 mg/mL oral solution: 50 mg/mL parenteral solution (IM).
Dosage:
Initial dosage: 10 mg bid. Titrate as needed to max of 250 mg/day in divided doses.
Maintenance: 50-100 mg/day.
Acute agitation: 12.5-50 mg IM q4-6h prn.
Elderly: 5-25 mg/day.
Potency (equivalent to 100 mg chlorpromazine): 12.5 mg.
Metabolism: Hepatic metabolism to active metabolite. Half-life 5-15 hours.
Therapeutic Level: Not established.
Clinical Guidelines: Loxapine may be associated with a higher risk of seizure than other high- and mid-potency agents. Concurrent use with medications that lower the seizure threshold should be avoided.

Molindone (Moban)

Class: Dihydroindolones
Preparations: 5, 10, 25, 100 mg tablets; 20 mg/mL conc. (PO)
Dosage:
Initial: 15-20 mg tid. Titrate to 10-40 mg tid-qid (max 225 mg/day)
Maintenance: 50-100 mg/day
Potency (equivalent to 100 mg chlorpromazine): 10 mg
Metabolism: Hepatic metabolism, half-life 10–20 hours.
Therapeutic Level: Not established
Clinical Guidelines: Studies suggest molindone is associated with less weight gain, amenorrhea, and impotence than other typical antipsychotics. Molindone appears less likely to cause seizures than other antipsychotics.

Perphenazine (Trilafon)

Class: Piperazine.
Preparations: 2, 4, 8, 16 mg tablets; 16 mg/5 mL oral solution; 5 mg/mL parenteral solution (IM).
Dosage:
  Initial: 4-8 mg tid, titrate to 8-16 mg bid-tid (max 64 mg/day).
  Maintenance: 4-40 mg/day.
  Acute agitation: 5-10 mg IM q 6h. prn (max 30 mg/day).
Potency (equivalent to 100 mg chlorpromazine): 10 mg.
Metabolism: Hepatic metabolism, half-life 10-20 hours.
Therapeutic Level: Not established.
Clinical Guidelines: Perphenazine has antiemetic properties.

References, see page 102.

Low-Potency Antipsychotics

Side-Effect Profile: High potentiation of anticholinergic, antihistamine, antiadrenergic agents. Orthostatic hypotension (moderate), sedation (high), anticholinergic (moderate), extrapyramidal symptoms (low). Neuroleptic malignant syndrome, tardive dyskinesia, and dystonic reactions are possible. Higher risk than most other antipsychotics for ECG changes (including T-wave changes), jaundice, decreased libido, and retrograde ejaculation.

Chlorpromazine (Thorazine)

Class: Aliphatic Phenothiazine.
Preparations:
Tablets: 10, 25, 50, 100, 200 mg; Slow-release capsules: 30, 75, 100, 200, 300 mg. Oral liquid preparations: 30 mg/mL and 100 mg/mL conc; 10 mg/5 mL syrup. Parenteral injection: 25 mg/mL (IM). Suppositories: 25, 100 mg (PR).
Dosage:

- **Initial:** 10-50 mg PO bid-qid, titrate to 200-800 mg/day in divided doses (max 2000 mg/day).
- **Acute agitation**: 25-50 mg IM q 4-6h.
- **Maintenance:** 200-800 mg/day.
- **Elderly:** Not recommended due to orthostatic hypotension.

Potency (equivalent to 100 mg chlorpromazine): 100 mg.
Metabolism: Hepatic metabolism to many metabolites.
Therapeutic Level: Not useful due to many active metabolites.
Major Safety Concerns:
Higher risk than most other typical antipsychotics for seizure, jaundice, photosensitivity, skin discoloration (bluish), and granular deposits in lens and cornea. Prolongation of QT and PR intervals, blunting of T-waves, ST segment depression can occur. Associated with a high incidence of hypotensive and anticholinergic side effects. Chlorpromazine has high lethality in overdose. It has a higher risk than many other antipsychotics for life-threatening agranulocytosis. Use chlorpromazine with caution in patients with a history of cardiovascular, liver, or renal disease. Avoid use in pregnancy (especially in first trimester).
Clinical Guidelines:
Can be used for treatment of nausea or vomiting (10-25 mg po qid; 25 mg IM qid; 100 mg suppository tid) and intractable hiccups (25-50 mg qid).

Mesoridazine (Serentil)

Class: Piperidine
Preparations: 10-, 25-, 50-, 100-mg tablets; 25 mg/mL oral solution; 25 mg/mL parenteral solution (IM).

Dosage:

Initial: 25-50 mg po tid. Titrate to 300 mg/day (max 400 mg/day).
Acute agitation: 25-50 mg IM. Dose may be repeated q 4-6 hour.
Maintenance: 100-400 mg/day.
Elderly: Avoid because of hypotension risk.

Potency (equivalent to 100 mg chlorpromazine): 50 mg.
Metabolism: Hepatic metabolism to many metabolites. Half-life 24-48 hours.
Therapeutic Level: Not established.
Major Safety Concerns: Because of its association with QT prolongation and subsequent increased risk for fatal arrhythmias, mesoridazine is reserved for only those patients who have not responded to other antipsychotic agents.

Thioridazine (Mellaril)

Class: Piperidine
Preparations: 10, 15, 25, 50, 100, 150, 200 mg tablets; 5 mg/mL, 30 mg/mL and 100 mg/mL oral solution.
Dosage:

Initial dosage: 25-100 mg tid; titrate to 100-400 mg bid (max 800 mg/day)
Maintenance: 200-800 mg/day; never exceed 800 mg/day No IM form available.
Elderly: avoid because of hypotension risk.

Potency (equivalent to 100 mg chlorpromazine): 100 mg.
Metabolism: Hepatic metabolism to active metabolites including mesoridazine, half-life 10-20 hours.
Therapeutic Level: Not established.
Major Safety Concerns: Because of its association with significant QT prolongation and subsequent increased risk for fatal arrhythmias, thioridazine is reserved for only those patients who have not responded to other antipsychotic agents. Permanent pigmentation of retina and potential blindness occurs with doses above 800 mg/day. Life-threatening agranulocytosis rarely occurs. Retrograde ejaculation occurs more frequently with thioridazine.

References, see page 102.

Anxiolytics

Anxiolytic medications are used for the treatment of anxiety. Some have shown efficacy in the treatment of specific anxiety disorders. Antidepressants are also used in the treatment of anxiety disorders.

Benzodiazepines

I. Indications

A. Benzodiazepines are used for the treatment of specific anxiety disorders, such as Panic Disorder, Social Phobia, Generalized Anxiety Disorder, and Adjustment Disorder with Anxious Mood (anxiety due to a specific stressful life event). All anxiolytic benzodiazepines can cause sedation.

II. Pharmacology

A. Benzodiazepines bind to benzodiazepine receptor sites, which are part of the GABA receptor. Benzodiazepine binding facilitates the action of GABA at the GABA receptor complex, which surrounds a chloride ion channel. GABA binding causes chloride influx into the neuron, with subsequent neuroinhibition.

B. The benzodiazepines differ in their absorption rates, lipid solubility, metabolism and half-lives. These factors will affect onset of action, length of action, drug interactions and side-effect profile.

C. The long half-life of diazepam, chlordiazepoxide, clorazepate, halazepam and prazepam (>100 hrs) is due to the active metabolite desmethyl-diazepam.

D. Most benzodiazepines are metabolized via the microsomal cytochrome P450 system in the liver. Hepatic metabolism involves discreet families of isozymes within the cytochrome system and most benzodiazepines are metabolized by the 3A3/4 isoenzyme family. Notable exceptions to this are lorazepam, oxazepam, temazepam and clonazepam.

III. Clinical Guidelines

A. Non-psychiatric causes of anxiety, including medical disorders, medications and substances of abuse should be excluded before beginning benzodiazepine treatment.

B. Choosing a benzodiazepine should be based on the patient's past response to medication, family history of medication response, medical conditions, current medications (drug interactions), and whether or not to choose a long half-life or short half-life drug. Long half-life drugs can be given less frequently, and they have less serum fluctuation and less severe withdrawal. These agents have a higher potential for drug accumulation and daytime sedation.

C. The initial dosage should be low and titrated up as necessary, especially when using long half-life drugs, since these may accumulate with multiple dosing over several days. The therapeutic dose for benzodiazepines is far below the lethal dose. Long-term use of benzodiazepines is associated with tolerance and dependence. Continued use of benzodiazepines for more than 3 weeks is associated with tolerance, dependence and a withdrawal syndrome.

1. Tolerance develops most readily to the sedative side effect of benzodiazepines.
2. Cross-tolerance may develop between benzodiazepines and other sedative hypnotic drugs, including alcohol.
3. Withdrawal symptoms include heightened anxiety, tremor, shakiness, muscle twitching, sweating, insomnia, tachycardia, hypertension with postural hypotension, and seizures.

D. Avoidance of an abstinence syndrome requires gradual tapering upon discontinuation. One-fourth of the dose per week is a good general guideline.

IV. Adverse Drug Reactions

A. Side Effects: The most common side effect is sedation. Dizziness, ataxia and impaired fine motor coordination can also occur. Some patients complain of cognitive impairment.

B. Anterograde amnesia has been reported, especially with benzodiazepines that reach peak levels quickly.

C. Respiratory depression is rarely an issue even in patients who overdose on benzodiazepines alone. However, patients who overdose with benzodiazepines and other sedative-hypnotics (commonly alcohol) may experience respiratory depression. Patients with compromised pulmonary function are more sensitive to this effect and even therapeutic doses may cause respiratory impairment.

D. Diazepam (Valium) and chlordiazepoxide (Librium) should not be used in patients with hepatic dysfunction because their metabolism will be impaired and toxicity risk increases.

E. Clonazepam should be avoided in patients with renal dysfunction because its metabolism will be impaired and the risk of toxicity will be high.

V. Drug Interactions

A. The concomitant use of benzodiazepines and other CNS depressant agents, including sedative-hypnotics, will enhance sedation and increase the risk of respiratory depression. Alcohol use should be limited.

B. Most benzodiazepines are metabolized via the liver enzyme CYP3A4; therefore, any other drug also metabolized via this pathway may increase the level of the benzodiazepine (except lorazepam, oxazepam, temazepam and clonazepam). Other agents that increase benzodiazepine levels include cimetidine, fluoxetine, ketoconazole, metoprolol, propranolol, estrogens, alcohol, erythromycin, disulfiram, valproic acid, nefazodone, and isoniazid. Benzodiazepine levels may be decreased by carbamazepine, rifampin (enzyme induction), and antacids (absorption).

References, see page 102.

Anxiolytic Benzodiazepines

Alprazolam (Xanax)

Indications: Panic Disorder, Social Phobia. Can be used in Generalized Anxiety Disorder (GAD) and Adjustment Disorder with Anxious Mood.
Preparations: 0.25, 0.5, 1, 2 mg tablets.
Dosage: 0.25-2 mg tid-qid.
Elderly: reduce dosage.
Half-Life: Up to 12 hrs.
The clinical duration of action is short despite moderate serum half-life.
Clinical Guidelines: Fast onset provides quick relief of acute anxiety. Alprazolam has a relatively short duration of action and multiple dosing throughout the day is required (some patients require as much as Qid dosing). It is associated with less sedation but a high incidence of inter-dose anxiety. Dependence and withdrawal are serious problems with this drug. Since SSRIs and other antidepressants are as effective in anxiety disorders, Alprazolam is no longer a first-line drug for the treatment of anxiety disorders.

Chlordiazepoxide (Librium, Libritabs)

Indications: Anxiety and alcohol withdrawal.
Preparations: 5, 10, 25 mg capsules.
Dosage:
Anxiety: 5-25 mg tid-qid.
Alcohol withdrawal: 25-50 mg every 2-4 hours (maximum 400 mg/day) prn.
Dose range: 10-100 mg/day.
Elderly: Avoid use
Half-Life: >100 hrs.
Clinical Guidelines: This drug will accumulate with multiple dosing. Because this drug is metabolized by P450 isoenzymes. Metabolism can be slowed in the elderly and patients with hepatic impairment. If used for anxiety, once-a-day dosing may be possible. Slower onset of action than Valium.

Clonazepam (Klonopin)

Indications: Approved as anticonvulsant. Used in Panic Disorder, Social Phobia and general anxiety. Useful in acute treatment of Mania.
Preparations: 0.5, 1, 2 mg tablets.
Dosage:
Anxiety: 0.25-6 mg Qod, in divided dose bid-tid.
Mania: 0.25-10 mg Qod, in divided dose bid-tid.
Elderly: 0.25-1.5 mg Qod.
Half-Life: 20-50 hrs. No active metabolites.

Clinical Guidelines: Rapid onset provides prompt relief. Clonazepam, with its long half-life, may be substituted for shorter acting benzodiazepines, such as alprazolam, in the treatment of benzodiazepine withdrawal and panic disorder. Its long half-life allows for once-a-day dosing.

Clorazepate (Tranxene)

Indications: Anxiety
Preparations: 3.75, 7.5, 11.25, 15, 22.5 mg tablets; 3.75, 7.5, 15 mg capsules
Pharmacology: Clorazepate is metabolized to desmethyldiazepam in the GI tract and absorbed in this active form.
Dosage:
- **Anxiety:** 7.5 mg tid or 15 mg qhs. Increase as needed.
- **Dose range:** 15-60 mg/day (maximum 90 mg/day).
- **Elderly:** Avoid use in the elderly.

Half-Life: >100 hrs.
Clinical Guidelines: This drug will accumulate with multiple dosing and over time. Because this drug is metabolized by P450 isoenzymes, metabolism can be slowed in the elderly and patients with hepatic impairment. If used for anxiety, once-a-day dosing may be possible.

Diazepam (Valium)

Indications: Anxiety, alcohol withdrawal.
Preparations: 2, 5, 10 mg tablets; 15 mg capsules (sustained release); 5 mg/mL solution for IV use. IM administration not recommended due to erratic incomplete absorption.
Dosage:
- **Anxiety:** 2-40 mg/day divided bid-tid.
- **Alcohol withdrawal:** 5-10 mg q 2-4 hr prn withdrawal signs for first 24 hrs, then slow taper. Maximum of 60 mg/day.
- **Dose range:** 2-60 mg/day.
- **Elderly:** Use with caution because metabolism is significantly delayed.

Half-Life: 100 hrs.
Clinical Guidelines: Diazepam is the most rapidly absorbed benzodiazepine. Due to its long half-life, it may accumulate with multiple dosing. Because this drug is metabolized by P450 isoenzymes, metabolism can be slowed in the elderly and patients with hepatic impairment. If used for anxiety, once-a-day dosing may be possible.

Halazepam (Paxipam)

Indications: Anxiety.
Preparations: 20, 40 mg tablets.
Dosage:
- **Anxiety:** 20-80 mg/day (divided doses).

Dose range: 40-160 mg/day. Use with caution in elderly.

Half-Life: >100 hrs .

Clinical Guidelines: This medication has no unique advantages over other benzodiazepines that have long half-lives and are metabolized by P450 isoenzymes.

Lorazepam (Ativan)

Indications: Anxiety, alcohol withdrawal, and adjunct in the treatment of acute psychotic agitation.

Preparations: 0.5, 1, 2 mg tablets; 2 mg/mL, 4 mg/mL soln (IV, IM).

This is the only benzodiazepine available in IM form that has rapid, complete, predictable absorption.

Dosage:

Anxiety: 0.5-6 mg/day (divided doses).

Alcohol withdrawal: 0.5-2 mg q 2-4 hr prn signs of alcohol withdrawal; or 0.5-1.0 mg IM to initiate treatment. Maximum dose of 10 mg/day.

Elderly: Metabolism is not significantly affected by age; elderly may be more susceptible to side effects.

Half-Life: 15 hrs. No active metabolites

Clinical Guidelines: Metabolism is not P450 dependent and will only be affected when hepatic dysfunction is severe. The inactive glucuronide is renally excreted; it is the benzodiazepine of choice in patients with serious or multiple medical conditions. It is the only benzodiazepine available in IM form with rapid and complete absorption. Its metabolism is not affected by age. These properties make it ideal for alcohol withdrawal in a patient with liver dysfunction or who is elderly. Since the half-life is relatively short, accumulation with multiple dosing usually does not occur. The IM form is useful in rapid control of agitation, resulting from psychosis, or drug-induced agitation. It is also widely used on a PO basis as a prn adjunct to fixed doses of antipsychotic medication.

References, see page 102.

Non-Benzodiazepine Anxiolytics

Buspirone (BuSpar)

Category: Non-benzodiazepine, non-sedative hypnotic anxiolytic.
Mechanism: Serotonin 1A agonist.
Indications: Generalized Anxiety Disorder (GAD). May be used to augment antidepressant treatment of Major Depressive Disorder and Obsessive-Compulsive Disorder (OCD). Often useful in the treatment of aggression and agitation in dementia and in patients with developmental disabilities.
Preparations: 5, 10, 15 and 30 mg tablets (15 mg and 30 mg tablet is scored so that it can be either bisected or trisected).
Dosage:
  Initial Dosage: 7.5 mg bid, then increase by 5 mg every 2-3 days as tolerated.
  Dose Range: 30-60 mg/day (maximum 60 mg/day).
  Elderly: 15-60 mg/day.
  Antidepressant Augmentation: 15-60 mg/day if a patient has a suboptimal response to a 4-6 week trial of an antidepressant.
Half-Life: 2-11 hours. No active metabolites.
Side Effects: Dizziness, headache, GI distress, fatigue.
Clinical Guidelines: Buspirone lacks the sedation and dependence associated with benzodiazepines, and it causes less cognitive impairment than the benzodiazepines. It is less effective in patients who have taken benzodiazepines in the past because it lacks the euphoria and sedation that these patients may expect with anxiety relief. Unlike benzodiazepines, buspirone does not immediately relieve anxiety. Onset of action may take 2 weeks. The patient may be started on a benzodiazepine and buspirone for two weeks, followed by slow tapering of the benzodiazepine.

Hydroxyzine (Atarax, Vistaril)

Category: Antihistamine, mild anxiolytic.
Mechanism: Histamine receptor antagonist, mild anticholinergic activity.
Indications: Anxiety (short-term treatment), sometimes used to augment the sedative side effects of antipsychotics when given for acute agitation.
Preparations: 10, 25, 50, 100 mg tablets; 10 mg/5 mL syrup; 50 mg/mL solution (IM, not IV).
Dosage:
  Anxiety: 50-100 PO q 4-6 hrs.
  Acute agitation: 50-100 mg IM q 4-6 hrs.
Side Effects: Dry mouth, dizziness, drowsiness, tremor, thickening of bronchial secretions, hypotension, decreased motor coordination.
Drug Interactions: The sedative effect of hydroxyzine will be enhanced by the concomitant use of other sedative drugs. Similarly, the mild anticholinergic

properties may be enhanced if another medication with anticholinergic properties is also taken.

Clinical Guidelines: Hydroxyzine is not associated with dependence. It is a weak anxiolytic and only effective for short-term treatment of anxiety. It can be helpful as an adjunct to antipsychotic medications since it will potentiate the sedative side effects and reduce the risk of extrapyramidal side effects.

References, see page 102.

Benzodiazepine Hypnotics

Hypnotic medications are used for the treatment of insomnia. Choice of agent is determined by half-life. Short-acting hypnotics are best for the treatment of initial insomnia or difficulties with sleep onset. They are associated with less morning sedation. Long-acting agents are more useful for the treatment of late insomnia or difficulties in maintaining sleep. These agents are more likely to be associated with daytime sedation.

I. **Indications**. Insomnia.

II. **Pharmacology**

- **A.** The major difference between the anxiolytic and hypnotic benzodiazepines is the rate of absorption.
- **B.** Benzodiazepine hypnotics are rapidly absorbed from the GI tract and achieve peak serum levels quickly, resulting in rapid onset of sedation.

III. **Clinical Guidelines**

- **A.** Hypnotics are recommended for short-term use only. Insomnia treatment should include exercise, stress reduction, sleep hygiene, and caffeine avoidance.
- **B.** Prolonged use of benzodiazepines (generally greater than 3 weeks) is associated with tolerance, dependence and withdrawal syndromes.
- **C.** The choice of benzodiazepine hypnotic is usually dictated by the need for sleep onset or sleep maintenance, half-life, and drug interactions.

IV. **Adverse Drug Reactions**

- **A.** Daytime sedation or morning “hangover” is a major complaint when patients take hypnotics with long half-lives. Dizziness and ataxia may occur during the daytime or if the patient awakens during the night. Anterograde amnesia has been reported.
- **B.** Benzodiazepines may depress respiration at high doses. Patients with compromised pulmonary function are more sensitive to this effect.

V. **Drug Interactions**

- **A.** Other CNS depressant agents, including the sedative-hypnotics will enhance the sedative effect of hypnotic benzodiazepines. Alcohol use should also be determined.
- **B.** Since triazolam, estazolam, flurazepam and quazepam are metabolized via the liver enzyme, CYP3A4, concomitant use of other medications with similar metabolism will increase the half-life effect and potential for toxicity.

Flurazepam (Dalmane)

Indications: Insomnia.
Preparations: 15, 30 mg tablets.
Dosage: Insomnia: 15-30 mg qhs, less in elderly.
Half-Life: 100 hrs.
Clinical Guidelines: Fast onset is useful in treatment of early insomnia. Long duration is useful in treatment of late insomnia but may result in morning sedation. Shorter half-life medications are preferable to flurazepam.

Estazolam (ProSom)

Indications: Insomnia.
Preparations: 1, 2 mg tablets.
Dosage:
Insomnia: 1-2 mg qhs
Elderly: 0.5-1.0 mg qhs.
Half-Life: 17 hrs.
Clinical Guidelines: Fast onset of action is useful for treatment of early insomnia. Medium half-life should help patients stay asleep throughout the night. Estazolam offers no real advantage over temazepam (Restoril). More clinicians are familiar with the use of estazolam. Estazolam is not commonly used.

Quazepam (Doral)

Indications: Insomnia.
Preparations: 7.5, 15 mg tablets.
Dosage:
Insomnia: 7.5-30 mg qhs.
Elderly: 7.5 mg qhs.
Half-Life: 100 hrs.
Clinical Guidelines: Long duration of action may result in morning sedation. It has no unique properties; it is not commonly used.

Temazepam (Restoril)

Indication: Insomnia.
Preparations: 7.5, 15, 30 mg capsules.
Dosage: Insomnia: 7.5-30 mg qhs (less for elderly).
Half-Life: 10-12 hrs.
Clinical Guidelines: Short duration of action limits morning sedation.

Triazolam (Halcion)

Indication: Insomnia.
Preparations: 0.125, 0.25 mg tablets.
Dosage: Insomnia: 0.125-0.25 mg qhs. Reduce dosage in elderly.
Half-life: 2-3 hrs.
Clinical Guidelines: Ultra-short half-life results in minimal AM sedation. It is best for sleep initiation. Patients may report waking up after 3-4 hours when blood level drops. It is not recommended for patients who have trouble maintaining sleep throughout the night. Use should be limited to 10 days.

Non-Benzodiazepine Hypnotics

Zolpidem (Ambien)

Category: Non-benzodiazepine hypnotic.
Mechanism: Binds to the GABA receptor, but is a non-benzodiazepine.
Indications: Insomnia.
Preparations: 5, 10 mg tablets.
Dosage: 10 mg qhs (5.0 mg for elderly).
Half-Life: 2-3 hrs.
Side Effects: Dizziness, GI upset, nausea, vomiting. Anterograde amnesia and morning "hangover" occur at dosages.
Drug–Drug Interactions: Potentiation of other CNS depressants (eg, alcohol). Higher serum levels reported in patients with hepatic insufficiency, but not with renal insufficiency.
Clinical Guidelines: Zolpidem has a rapid onset. It is especially useful for initiating sleep. Zolpidem is not associated with dependence or withdrawal. Zolpidem is rated a pregnancy category B.

Zaleplon (Sonata)

Category: Non-benzodiazepine hypnotic.
Mechanism: Binds to the GABA receptor, but is a non-benzodiazepine.
Indications: Insomnia.
Preparations: 5-, 10-mg tablets.
Dosage: 10 mg qhs (5.0 mg for elderly).
Half-Life: 1 hr.
Side Effects: Dizziness, dyspepsia, and diarrhea.
Drug–Drug Interactions: Potentiation of other CNS depressants (eg, alcohol). Higher serum levels reported in patients with hepatic insufficiency, but not with moderate renal insufficiency. Cimetidine can increase serum levels.
Clinical Guidelines: Zaleplon has a rapid onset. It is especially useful for initiating sleep and is not associated with dependence or withdrawal. Because of its short half-life, a repeat dose may be given. It is rated pregnancy category

Diphenhydramine (Benadryl)

Category: Antihistamine.
Mechanism: Histamine receptor antagonist (sedation), acetylcholine receptor antagonist (extrapyramidal symptom control).
Indications: Mild insomnia, neuroleptic-induced extrapyramidal symptoms, antihistamine.
Preparations: 25, 50 mg tablets; 25, 50 mg capsules; 10 mg/mL and 50 mg/mL soln. (IM, IV), 12.5 mg/5 mL elixir (PO).

Dosage:
Insomnia: 50 mg PO qhs.
Extrapyramidal symptoms: 25-50 mg PO bid, for acute extrapyramidal. symptoms 25-50 mg IM or IV.
Half-Life: 1-4 hrs.
Side Effects: Dry mouth, dizziness, drowsiness, tremor, thickening of bronchial secretions, hypotension, decreased motor coordination, GI distress.
Interactions: Diphenhydramine has an additive effect when used with other sedatives and other medications with anticholinergic activity. May cause exacerbation of narrow angle glaucoma and prostatic hypertrophy. MAO inhibitor use is contraindicated within 2 weeks of diphenhydramine.
Clinical Guidelines: Diphenhydramine is a very weak sedative, and it is minimally effective as a hypnotic. It is non-addicting.

Chloral Hydrate (Somnote)

Category: Sedative-hypnotic.
Mechanism: CNS depression, specific mechanism is unknown.
Indications: Insomnia.
Preparations: 500 mg capsules.
Dosage: 500-1000 mg qhs (short-term only).
Half-Life: 8 hrs.
Side Effects: Nausea, vomiting, diarrhea, daytime sedation and impaired coordination.
Interactions: IV furosemide may cause flushing and labile blood pressure. Additive effects when given with other CNS depressants.
Clinical Guidelines: Tolerance and dependence regularly develop with consistent use. It is highly lethal in overdose and can cause hepatic and renal damage. Its use has decreased since benzodiazepines are equally effective and are much safer.

References, see page 102.

Barbiturates

Barbiturate use has diminished since the introduction of benzodiazepines due to their lower therapeutic index and high abuse potential.

I. **Indications**

A. There are very few psychiatric indications for barbiturates since benzodiazepines are safer and just as effective. The phenobarbital challenge test is also used to quantify sedative-hypnotic abuse in patients abusing multiple sedative hypnotics, including alcohol.

B. Given the availability of equally effective and safer benzodiazepines, it is difficult to justify the long-term use of barbiturates.

II. **Pharmacology**

A. Barbiturates bind to barbiturate receptor sites, which are part of the GABA receptor. Barbiturate binding facilitates the action of GABA at the GABA receptor complex, resulting in inhibition.

B. Barbiturates induce hepatic microsomal enzymes and may reduce levels of other medications with hepatic metabolism.

III. **Clinical Guidelines**

A. Continued use of barbiturates for more than 3-4 weeks is associated with tolerance, dependence and withdrawal syndrome.

1. Tolerance develops to the sedative side effects. Cross-tolerance between barbiturates and other sedative hypnotic drugs, including alcohol, may develop.
2. Withdrawal symptoms include: heightened anxiety, tremor, muscle twitching, sweating, insomnia, tachycardia, hypertension with postural hypotension and seizures.
3. The severity of withdrawal is determined by the rate of decreasing serum level. Faster rates of decline are associated with more sever withdrawal.

B. Avoidance of an abstinence syndrome requires gradual tapering upon discontinuation. A long half-life benzodiazepine (eg, clonazepam) helps to reduce the severity of withdrawal.

C. Barbiturates should not be used in pregnancy. Infants born to habituated mothers may have respiratory depression at birth and will go into withdrawal.

IV. **Adverse Drug Reactions**

A. The most common side effect is sedation and impaired concentration. Dizziness, ataxia and impaired fine motor coordination can also occur.

B. Barbiturates should not be used in patients with hepatic dysfunction since their metabolism will be impaired and toxicity may occur. Barbiturates are contraindicated in patients with acute intermittent porphyria since they may cause the production of porphyrins.

V. **Drug Interactions**

A. The concomitant use of benzodiazepines and CNS depressant agents, including sedative-hypnotics, will enhance sedation and increase the risk of respiratory depression. Alcohol use should be limited.

B. Barbiturates enhance the metabolism of a number of commonly used medications because they induce hepatic enzymes. Reduced effectiveness of these medications can occur. These include anticoagulants, tricyclic antidepressants, propranolol, carbamazepine, estrogen (oral contraceptives), corticosteroids, quinidine, and theophylline.

C. The effect of barbiturates on phenytoin metabolism is unpredictable, phenytoin levels should be monitored. Valproate inhibits barbiturate metabolism.

Amobarbital (Amytal)

Preparations: 30, 50, 100 mg tablets; 65, 200 mg capsules; 250 mg/5 mL, 500 mg/5 mL solution (IM, IV).

Dosage:

Sedation: 50-100 PO or IM.

Hypnosis: 50-200 mg IV (max 400 mg/day).

Half-life: 8-42 hrs.

Clinical Guidelines: Lorazepam has largely replaced the use of amobarbital for emergent control of psychotic agitation. The use of amobarbital in clinical diagnosis has also decreased.

Pentobarbital (Nembutal)

Preparations: 50, 100 mg capsules.

Dosage: 200 mg PO.

Half-Life: 15-48 hrs.

Pentobarbital Challenge Test: The pentobarbital challenge test is a useful method of quantifying the daily intake of sedative hypnotics so that patients can be detoxified. Patients are given 200 mg orally and after one hour, the level of intoxication is assessed. If no signs of intoxication, 100 mg is given, and the patient is reassessed after one hour. Repeat procedure every two hours until signs of intoxication occur (Nystagmus is the most sensitive sign and sleep is the most obvious sign). Maximum dose 600 mg. The dose required to show signs of intoxication is the equivalent dose to the daily habit of sedative hypnotics. Substitute a long half-life drug in divided doses and gradually taper by 10% per day.

References, see page 102.

Mood Stabilizers

Mood stabilizers are used for the treatment of mania, depression, and bipolar disorder and schizoaffective disorder. They are also used for the treatment of severe cyclothymia and unipolar depression. They can be helpful in the treatment of impulse control disorders, severe personality disorders, and behavioral disorders. Mood stabilizers include lithium, anticonvulsants, and calcium channel blockers.

Lithium Carbonate (Eskalith, Lithobid, Lithonate, Eskalith CR)

I. Indications

A. Lithium is effective in the treatment of the acute manic phase of bipolar disorder as well as maintenance treatment of bipolar disorder. It is more effective in the treatment of the manic episodes of bipolar disorder than in the depressed episodes. Antidepressants are often added to lithium when treating bipolar depressed patients. Antidepressant medication can trigger manic episodes in bipolar patients has been shown to enhance the risk of rapid cycling patterns.

B. Lithium is also used clinically for schizoaffective disorder and severe cyclothymia.

C. In depressed patients who have not responded to antidepressants, lithium augmentation may enhance response. Lithium augmentation may be a useful treatment strategy in some patients with schizophrenia that does not respond adequately to antipsychotics.

D. Lithium may be helpful in treating borderline personality disorder, certain impulse control disorders such as intermittent explosive disorder and behavioral disturbances.

II. Pharmacology

A. Lithium may act by blocking inositol-1-phosphatase in neurons with subsequent interruption of the phosphatidylinositol second messenger system.

B. Lithium is excreted by the kidneys. Impaired renal function or decreased fluid and salt intake can lead to toxicity. An age-related reduction in creatinine clearance will lead to reduced lithium clearance in the elderly. Lower doses and close monitoring are required in the elderly.

C. Preparations

1. Rapid absorption - Eskalith caps (300 mg), lithium carbonate caps and tabs (300 mg), Lithonate caps (300 mg), Lithotabs tabs (300 mg).
2. Slow release - Lithobid tabs (300 mg), Eskalith CR (450 mg).
3. Lithium citrate syrup: 8 mEq/5 mL (rapid absorption).

D. Half-Life: 20 hrs.

III. Clinical Guidelines

A. Lithium is the first-line drug in the treatment of bipolar disorder. Valproate may also be used. Approximately 30% of patients with bipolar disorder will not respond to lithium.

B. **Pre-Lithium Work-up:** Non-psychiatric causes of mood disorder or manic symptoms should be excluded before initiating lithium, including medical disorders, medications and substances of abuse. In the absence of clinical symptoms of a medical disorder, screening laboratory studies should be ordered to monitor the effects of lithium. These include a basic chemistry panel, thyroid function tests, CBC, and an EKG in patients who are over 40 years old or with pre-existing cardiac disease. In females of childbearing age, pregnancy should be excluded.

IV. Dosage and Administration

A. Lithium is given in divided doses. Bid dosing with a slow-release formula is recommended. The starting dose for most adults is 300 mg bid-tid. The average dose rage is 900-2100 mg/day.

B. Single daily dosing can be used if the daily dose is less than 1200 mg/day. Divided doses cause less GI upset and tremor.

C. Upward titration of lithium should occur until a serum level of 0.8-1.2 mEq/L is obtained. Some patients on long-term maintenance can be managed at lower serum levels between 0.5-0.8 mEq/L.

D. Serum lithium levels can be obtained after five days at any given dosage. Serum levels should be drawn 12 hours after the previous dose and are usually done in the morning before the AM dose. Serum levels should be monitored weekly for the first 1-2 months, then biweekly for another 2 months. A patient who has been stable on lithium for a year can be monitored every 3-4 months.

E. **Therapeutic Response:** Therapeutic effect may take 4-6 weeks. True prophylactic effect may take >2 months.

F. **Pregnancy and Lactation:** Pregnancy category D. Lithium should not be administered to pregnant women in the first trimester when it is associated with an increased incidence of birth defects, especially Ebstein's anomaly. After the first trimester, lithium treatment may be initiated on a risk-benefit basis. Breast feeding in contraindicated.

V. Adverse Drug Reactions

A. **Side Effects:** The most common side effects are GI distress, weight gain, fine tremor, and cognitive impairment ("fuzzy thinking"). Nausea, vomiting and tremor can be alleviated by dividing the dose, taking it with food or switching to a slow-release preparation. Small doses of propranolol (eg, 10 mg bid-tid) can also reduce or even eliminate tremor.

B. **Renal:** Polyuria with secondary polydipsia occurs in 20%. Lithium-induced diabetes insipidus may be treated with the diuretic amiloride (5-10 mg/day). Renal function should be monitored.

C. **Thyroid:** Hypothyroidism may occur, and it may be treated with levothyroxine. Monitor TSH several times per year.

D. **Cardiovascular:** Cardiovascular side effects include T-wave flattening or inversion and, rarely, arrhythmias which usually require discontinuation. Edema may respond to spironolactone 50 mg/day, or a reduction of the lithium dose.

E. **Dermatological:** Side effects include rash and acne. Both problems may respond to dose reductions, and acne can be treated with benzoyl peroxide or topical antibiotics. Lithium can induce or exacerbate psoriasis, which usually responds to discontinuation of lithium. Alopecia will also respond to discontinuation of lithium.

F. **Hematologic:** A benign leukocytosis can occur with lithium. No treatment is indicated, but infection should be excluded.

G. **Neurologic:** Muscle weakness, fasciculations, clonic movements, slurred speech and headaches have been reported. These symptoms may subside with time.

H. **Lithium Toxicity**

1. Reduced fluid intake, increased fluid loss (excessive sweating) or reduced salt intake may lead to toxicity.
2. Symptoms of lithium toxicity include nausea, vomiting, and diarrhea, coarse tremor (in contrast to the fine tremor seen at therapeutic doses). Ataxia, headache, slurred speech, confusion, arrhythmias may also occur.
3. Mild-to-moderate toxicity occurs at 1.5-2.0 mEq/L. Severe toxicity occurs at levels over 2.5 mEq/L. Death may occur at levels >4.0 mEq/L.

VI. **Drug Interactions**

A. The most common cause of drug interactions is a change in the renal clearance of lithium.

B. Medications that decrease lithium levels include:

1. Xanthines (theophylline, aminophylline, caffeine).
2. Increased dietary sodium and sodium bicarbonate (antacids).
3. Carbonic anhydrase inhibitors (acetazolamide).
4. Osmotic diuretics (mannitol).

C. Medications that increase lithium levels and increase the risk of toxicity include the following:

1. Potassium sparing diuretics (spironolactone), loop diuretics (furosemide), NSAIDS.

D. Neurotoxicity is a frequent consequence of lithium toxicity, and a number of medications will enhance the risk of lithium neurotoxicity. These medication include methyldopa, typical antipsychotics, carbamazepine, phenytoin calcium channel blockers. Close monitoring for symptoms of neurotoxicity is recommended. These symptoms include tremor, disorientation, confusion, ataxia, and headaches.

E. The action of neuromuscular-blocking agents, especially succinylcholine, will be prolonged by lithium. Prolonged recovery from electroconvulsive therapy, often requiring ventilatory assistance, may occur. Lithium should be discontinued prior to electroconvulsive therapy.

References, see page 102.

Anticonvulsants

Anticonvulsants are primarily used for the treatment of bipolar disorder. Increasingly; they are replacing lithium as a first-line treatment in acute mania and the long-term prophylaxis of mood episodes in bipolar disorder. The prophylactic action of anticonvulsants in bipolar disorder is based on the theory of kindling, whereby repeated subthreshold stimulation of a neuron will eventually result in the spontaneous firing of the neuron. Anticonvulsants are more effective than lithium in the treatment of rapid-cycling and mixed bipolar states, impulse control disorders, treatment resistant depressive disorder, borderline personality disorder and other disorders with impulsive, unpredictable and/or aggressive behavior. Some newer anticonvulsants such as pregabalin are being studied primarily for the treatment of anxiety disorders.

Carbamazepine (Tegretol)

I. **Indications**

   A. Carbamazepine is used for the treatment of the acute manic phase of bipolar disorder and for maintenance treatment of bipolar disorder. It may be used alone or in combination with lithium. It is more effective than lithium in treating rapid-cycling bipolar disorder and mixed episodes.

   B. Carbamazepine is more effective in the treatment and prophylaxis of manic episodes than the depressed episodes of bipolar disorder. When treating the depressed episode of bipolar disorder with an antidepressant, it is necessary to maintain carbamazepine treatment to prevent an antidepressant-induced manic episode or rapid cycling.

   C. Carbamazepine is also used in the treatment of cyclothymia and schizoaffective disorder. It is frequently used with antipsychotics and/or lithium in schizoaffective disorder.

   D. Carbamazepine augmentation of antipsychotic medication can be useful in patient with schizophrenia when there is inadequate response to antipsychotics alone. It is particularly helpful for aggressive or impulsive behavior.

   E. Carbamazepine may be helpful in treating certain impulse control disorders, such as those seen in patients with developmental disabilities. It may also be helpful to reduce symptoms of impulsivity and affective instability in patients with severe personality disorders.

   F. Augmentation of antidepressant treatment with carbamazepine might be helpful in depressed patients who are treatment-resistant.

II. **Pharmacology**

   A. The mechanism of carbamazepine in psychiatric disorders is unknown.

   B. Carbamazepine is metabolized by the liver (CYP3A4) and its metabolites are excreted renally. It will induce it's own metabolism and serum levels tend to decrease with time, requiring an increase in the dosage. Initially, the half-life can be 25-65 hours. After several weeks, the serum half-life can decrease to 12-17 hours.

   C. Preparations: 100, 200 mg tablets; 100 mg/5 ml oral suspension.

III. Clinical Guidelines

A. Pre-Carbamazepine Work-Up

1. Non-psychiatric causes of mood disorder or manic symptoms, including medical disorders, medications and substances of abuse should be excluded before beginning carbamazepine treatment.
2. Screening labs should include a basic chemistry panel, CBC and an EKG in patients over 40 years old or with pre-existing cardiac disease. Pregnancy should be excluded in women of childbearing age.

B. Carbamazepine should not be given to patients with pre-existing liver, cardiac, or hematological disease. It is not recommended for patients with renal dysfunction because it has active metabolites that are renally excreted.

C. If carbamazepine is used in patients who have not responded to lithium, the carbamazepine should be added to the drug regimen. If the patient responds, the lithium should be withdrawn in an attempt to manage the patient with a single mood stabilizer.

D. Dosage and Administration

1. Starting dose is 200 mg Bid. The average dose range is 600–1200 mg/day. The dosage should be reduced by one-half in the elderly.
2. Dosage increases, especially when initiating treatment, can cause proportionally larger increases in serum level; therefore, the dosage should not be increased by more than 200 mg/day at a time.
3. Carbamazepine should be titrated to a serum level of 8-12 µg/mL. Serum carbamazepine levels should be obtained after five days at any given dosage. Serum levels should be drawn 12 hours after the previous dose, usually in the morning before the AM dose.
4. Serum levels should be monitored weekly for the first 1-2 months, then biweekly for another 2 months. Carbamazepine will induce its own metabolism, decreasing the serum level. The dosage may need to be increased in order to maintain a serum level within therapeutic range after initial stabilization. Frequent monitoring of serum level is recommended during the first three months of treatment.
5. A patient who has been stable on carbamazepine for a year can be monitored every 3-4 months. CBC and liver function, electrolytes and renal function should be checked after one month, then quarterly for the first year.

E. Therapeutic Response: Therapeutic effect may take 2-4 weeks.

F. Pregnancy and Lactation: Pregnancy category C. Carbamazepine is contraindicated during pregnancy or lactation. There may be an association between use of carbamazepine in pregnancy and congenital malformations, including spina bifida.

IV. Adverse Drug Effects

A. Side Effects: The most common side effects are GI complaints (nausea, vomiting, constipation, diarrhea, loss of appetite) and CNS complaints (sedation, dizziness, ataxia, confusion). These can be prevented or significantly reduced by increasing the daily dosage slowly.

B. Hematological

1. Carbamazepine causes life-threatening thrombocytopenia, agranulocytosis, and aplastic anemia in 0.005% of patients. Patients should contact their physician immediately with any signs of infection (fever, sore throat) or bleeding abnormality (easy bruising, petechiae, pallor).

A CBC should be drawn immediately. Carbamazepine should be discontinued if the WBC declines to less than 3000 mm^3, absolute neutrophil count <1500 mm^3 or platelet count decreases to <100,000 per mm^3.

2. Transient and minor decreases in blood cell indices can occur in the early phase of treatment and do not warrant discontinuation of carbamazepine.

C. Hepatic: Hepatitis and cholestatic jaundice may occur. The medication should be discontinued immediately.

D. Dermatological: Rash and urticaria are relatively common. Photosensitivity reactions may rarely occur. Potentially dangerous, but extremely rare, dermatological side effects include exfoliative dermatitis, toxic epidermal necrolysis and Stevens-Johnson syndrome, requiring immediate discontinuation of the drug.

E. Anticholinergic: Carbamazepine has mild anticholinergic activity and may exacerbate glaucoma and prostatic hypertrophy.

F. Cardiac: Uncommon side effects include AV conduction defects, arrhythmias, and congestive heart failure.

G. Metabolic/Endocrine: SIADH with hyponatremia has been reported.

H. Genitourinary: Urinary frequency, urinary retention, azotemia, renal failure and impotence are uncommon.

I. Toxicity: Signs of toxicity include confusion, stupor, motor restlessness, ataxia, mydriasis, muscle twitching, tremor, athetoid movements, nystagmus, abnormal reflexes, oliguria, nausea and vomiting. Cardiac arrhythmias do not generally occur unless very large doses are ingested.

V. Drug Interactions

A. The following medications inhibit the metabolism of carbamazepine with resultant increase in serum levels and neurotoxicity:

1. Verapamil and diltiazem.
2. Danazol.
3. Erythromycin.
4. Fluoxetine.
5. Cimetidine (transient effect). Not seen with ranitidine or famotidine.
6. Isoniazid.
7. Ketoconazole.
8. Loratadine.

B. The following medications cause cytochrome P450 enzyme induction and decreased carbamazepine levels:

1. Rifampin.
2. Cisplatin.

C. Anticonvulsant Interactions with Carbamazepine

1. Phenobarbital will lower carbamazepine levels due to microsomal enzyme induction.
2. When phenytoin and carbamazepine are given at the same time, the levels of both drugs may be decreased.
3. Decreased ethosuximide levels due to cytochrome P450 enzyme induction.
4. Felbamate can decrease carbamazepine levels but increase the active metabolite, which has been implicated in toxicity.

5. Lamotrigine and valproate can increase the active metabolite. Patients may have signs of toxicity with normal carbamazepine levels. Carbamazepine will cause decreased valproate levels.

D. Carbamazepine will induce hepatic microsomal enzymes and enhance the metabolism, decrease serum levels and decrease the effectiveness of the following medications:
1. Acetaminophen (may also enhance hepatotoxicity in overdose).
2. Clozapine and haloperidol.
3. Benzodiazepines (especially alprazolam, triazolam).
4. Oral contraceptives.
5. Corticosteroids.
6. Cyclosporine.
7. Doxycycline.
8. Mebendazole.
9. Methadone.
10. Theophylline (can also decrease carbamazepine levels).
11. Thyroid supplements (may mask compensatory increases in TSH).
12. Valproate.
13. Warfarin.

E. Diuretics should be used with caution since hyponatremia can occur with carbamazepine alone.

F. A minimum 14-day washout should elapse before beginning an MAOI due to the molecular similarity between tricyclic antidepressants and carbamazepine.

Valproic Acid (Depakene) and Divalproex (Depakote, Depakote ER)

I. Indications

A. Valproate may be used with lithium or alone in bipolar disorder and schizoaffective disorder.

B. It is more effective in rapid cycling and mixed episode bipolar disorder than lithium.

C. Recent evidence suggests that valproate may be more effective in treating depressive episodes compared to lithium and carbamazepine. However, it remains more effective in the treatment prophylaxis of manic episodes than the depressed episodes of bipolar disorder.

D. Valproate augmentation may be a useful treatment strategy in patients with schizophrenia who have not responded adequately to antipsychotics alone. It is particularly helpful in patients with aggressive or impulsive behavior.

E. There have been reports that it may be helpful in treating certain impulse control disorders such as intermittent explosive disorder and aggressive, impulsive behavior in patients with developmental disabilities. It may also be helpful to reduce symptoms of impulsivity and affective instability in patients with severe personality disorders.

II. Psychopharmacology

A. Valproate causes decreased GABA metabolism with secondary increased CNS GABA concentrations. Valproate may also impact signal transduction through actions on protein kinase C. It is unknown if these mechanisms are involved in the treatment of psychiatric disorders.

B. The average half-life is 8-10 hours, making bid-tid dosing necessary.

C. Pharmacokinetics and Metabolism of Valproate

1. Valproate is metabolized by the liver via mitochondrial beta-oxidation, glucuronidation and the P450 microsomal system. Unlike many other psychotropic medications, cytochrome P450 is relatively unimportant in valproate metabolism and medications that affect P450 have little effect on valproate serum levels.
2. The relationship between dose and blood level at the higher end of the therapeutic range is less helpful. Serum levels can be helpful to establish minimum dosages at the low end of the therapeutic range, but at higher levels, it is probably more important to monitor clinical symptoms of toxicity and side effects.
3. Valproate is highly protein bound and, at higher concentrations, this system becomes saturated and there is more unbound drug available. This actually enhances the metabolism of the drug and lowers the serum concentration.
4. Decreased protein binding (higher serum levels) is seen in the elderly and patients with hepatic and renal disease. These patients are at greater risk for toxicity.

D. Preparations: Valproic acid – 250 mg capsules; 250 mg/5 mL oral susp.
Divalproex – 125 mg, 250 mg, 500 mg tablets.
Extended release (Depakote ER) – 500 mg tablets

III. Clinical Guidelines

A. Valproate may be used as a first-line drug in the treatment of bipolar disorder, especially in patients with rapid cycling bipolar disorder or mixed mood episode.

B. Pre-Valproate Work-Up

1. Non-psychiatric causes of mood disorder or manic symptoms, including medical disorders, medications and substances of abuse should be excluded before beginning valproate treatment.
2. Screening laboratory exams should include liver function tests and a CBC. In females of childbearing age, pregnancy should be excluded.

C. Valproate should not be given to patients with pre-existing hepatic or hematological disease.

D. Dosage and Administration

1. Initiation of treatment begins with 20 mg/kg/day or approximately 500 mg tid or 750 mg Bid, then titrating up or down, depending on the serum level. The average daily dose is between 1500 and 2500 mg/day. The extended release formulation allows once daily dosing and the bioavailability is 80-90 % compared to Depakote. The elderly will require doses nearly half that of younger adults.
2. A serum level of 50-125 µg/mL is usually adequate for symptom relief. Serum levels in the low range are more accurate and more clinically useful compared to the high end of the therapeutic range. Patients can often tolerate levels up to 150 µg/mL.
3. Serum valproate levels can be obtained after 3 days at any given dosage. Serum levels should be drawn 12 hours after the previous dose and are usually done in the morning before the AM dose.

4. Serum levels should be monitored weekly for the first 1-2 months, then biweekly for another 2 months. A patient who has been stable for a year can be monitored every 3-4 months. CBC and liver function tests should be drawn after one month then quarterly for the first year.

E. **Therapeutic Response:** Therapeutic effect may take 2-4 weeks.

F. **Pregnancy and Lactation:** Pregnancy Category D. Valproate should not be used in pregnancy or breast-feeding. An increased incidence of neural tube defects and other birth defects has been reported. Fatal clotting abnormalities and hepatic failure have occurred in infants.

IV. **Adverse Drug Reactions**

A. **Side Effects:** The most common side effects are sedation, dizziness, nausea and vomiting (divalproex has lower incidence of GI side effects). GI side effects tend to decrease over time, especially if the drug is taken with food.

B. **Pancreatitis:** A rare but serious adverse effect is pancreatitis. It usually occurs early in treatment.

C. **Hepatic**

1. Hepatitis, which can be fatal, occurs in 0.0005% of patients. It is most common in children. Symptoms include lethargy and malaise, vomiting, loss of appetite, jaundice and weakness, usually occurring in the first 6 months of treatment. Valproate should be discontinued immediately if hepatitis is suspected.
2. A transient early increase in liver enzymes may occur in up to 25% of patients but does not predict the development of hepatitis. Close monitoring of liver enzymes is important to distinguish the benign temporary increase in hepatic enzymes from more dangerous hepatitis.

D. **Hematological:** Thrombocytopenia and platelet dysfunction can occur with secondary bleeding abnormalities.

E. **Neurological:** Tremor, ataxia, headache, insomnia, agitation

F. **Other GI side effects:** Changes in appetite and weight, diarrhea or constipation.

G. **Dermatological:** Alopecia, maculopapular rash.

H. **Overdose:** Symptoms of toxicity/overdose include somnolence, heart block and coma.

I. **Urea Cycle Disorders:** Hyperammonemic encephalopathy, sometimes fatal, can occur in patients with urea cycle disorders. These disorders are uncommon genetic diseases such as ornithine transcarbamlyase deficiency.

V. **Drug Interactions**

A. The following medications inhibit the metabolism of valproate with resultant increases in serum levels and increased potential for toxicity:

1. Aspirin inhibits metabolism and decreases bound fraction
2. Felbamate
3. Rifampin

B. **Anticonvulsant Interactions**

1. Phenobarbital causes non-P450 enzyme induction and lowers valproate levels. Valproate inhibits phenobarbital metabolism.
2. Phenytoin causes non-P450 enzyme induction and lowers valproate levels. Levels of both drugs should be monitored.
3. Carbamazepine causes non-P450 enzyme induction and lowers valproate levels. Valproate may not affect carbamazepine levels but will

increase serum levels of the active metabolite. Patients should be monitored for symptoms of carbamazepine toxicity.

4. Valproate inhibits the metabolism of lamotrigine and ethosuximide.
5. The combination of valproate and clonazepam has been reported to cause absence seizures.

C. Other Interactions

1. Valproate inhibits the metabolism of diazepam, resulting in increased levels.
2. Valproate inhibits the metabolism of AZT.
3. Valproate can displace warfarin from protein binding. Careful monitoring of clotting times is recommended.

Gabapentin (Neurontin)

I. Indications

A. While initial studies with gabapentin showed promise in the treatment of cyclic affective illness, data does not currently indicate significant efficacy for this medication in monotherapy or as an adjunctive agent.

B. Gabapentin is still often used as an adjunctive agent in cyclic affective illness and other psychiatric conditions to alleviate anxiety and assist with sleep and low-grade iritability.

II. Pharmacology

A. Gabapentin is chemically related to the neurotransmitter GABA, but it does not act on GABA receptors. It is not converted into GABA and does not effect GABA metabolism or reuptake. The mechanism in psychiatric disorders is unknown.

B. Gabapentin is excreted renally in an unchanged state. Reduced clearance of gabapentin with age is largely caused by reduced renal function.

C. Half-life: 5-7 hrs.

D. Preparations: 100, 300, 400, 600, 800 mg capsules

III. Clinical Guidelines

A. Pre-Gabapentin Work-Up: Non-psychiatric causes of mood disorder or mood symptoms (mania and depression), including medical disorders, medications and substances of abuse should be excluded before beginning gabapentin treatment. Screening laboratory exams should be ordered to monitor renal function. In females of childbearing age, pregnancy should be excluded.

B. Dosage and Administration

1. Starting dose can be 300 mg qhs, then increasing by 300 mg each day. The average daily dose is between 900 and 1800 mg/day, but doses up to 2400 have been used.
2. Monitoring of serum levels is not necessary. There is no information available regarding a therapeutic window.
3. Significantly lower doses should be given to patients with impaired renal function or reduced creatinine clearance.

C. Therapeutic Response: 2-4 weeks

D. Pregnancy and Lactation: Pregnancy category C. There are no controlled studies in pregnant women. Gabapentin should be avoided during the first trimester. Use after the first trimester must be on a risk-benefit basis. Mothers should be encouraged not to breast feed since the risks are unknown.

IV. **Adverse Drug Reactions**

A. **Side Effects**

1. The most common side effects are somnolence, fatigue, ataxia, nausea and vomiting and dizziness.
2. **Metabolic:** Weight gain, weight loss, edema.
3. **Cardiovascular:** Hypertension.
4. **GI:** Loss of appetite, increased appetite, dyspepsia, flatulence, gingivitis.
5. **Hematological:** Easy bruising.
6. **Musculoskeletal:** Arthralgia.
7. **CNS:** Nystagmus, tremor, diplopia, blurred vision.
8. **Psychiatric:** Anxiety, irritability, hostility, agitation, depression.

V. **Drug Interactions**

A. There are no interactions with other anticonvulsants.

B. Gabapentin has reduced absorption with antacids, and it should be taken at least 2 hours after antacid administration.

Lamotrigine (Lamictal)

I. **Indications**

A. Lamotrigine has efficacy in the treatment of bipolar depression as an adjunctive agent or as monotherapy. It has also been shown to decrease relapse to depression in stable bipolar patients by itself. Its efficacy in the treatment of bipolar mania or rapid cycling is not supported by current data. It is recommended that lamotrigine be used primarily as an adjunctive agent due to lack of proven efficacy in the treatment or prevention of mania.

B. It is more effective in depression compared to other mood stabilizers, prompting use in treatment-resistant unipolar depression. Controlled studies are currently underway.

II. **Pharmacology**

A. The mechanism of action is unknown. It may have an effect on sodium channels that modulate release of glutamate and aspartate. It also has a weak inhibitory effect on 5-HT_3 receptors.

B. Lamotrigine is hepatically metabolized via glucuronidation with subsequent renal excretion of the inactive glucuronide.

C. **Half-Life:** 25 hours.

D. **Preparations:** 25, 100, 150, 200 mg scored tablets.

III. **Clinical Guidelines**

A. Non-psychiatric causes of mood disorder or mood symptoms (mania and depression), including medical disorders, medications and substances of abuse should be excluded before beginning lamotrigine treatment.

B. Screening laboratory exams should be ordered to monitor renal and hepatic function. In females of childbearing age, pregnancy should be excluded.

C. **Dosage and Administration**
   1. The initial dose is 25 mg/day increased weekly to 50 mg/day, 100mg/day, and then 200 mg/day.
   2. In patients taking valproate, the dosage is 25 mg every other day for two weeks, then 25 mg per day for the next two weeks. In patients taking phenytoin, carbamazepine, phenobarbital or primidone without valproate, the dosage is 50 mg/day for two weeks, then 50 mg bid for the next two weeks. Average daily dose: 100-200 mg/day. Antidepressant effect may require up to 400 mg/day which may be given in a divided dose.
   3. Renal dysfunction does not markedly affect the half-life of lamotrigine. However, caution should be used when treating patients with renal disease since there is very little data in this population.

D. **Therapeutic Response:** Clinical effect: 2-4 weeks.

E. **Pregnancy and Lactation**
   1. Pregnancy category C. There are no controlled studies in pregnant women. Lamotrigine should be avoided during the first trimester.
   2. Use after the first trimester must be on a risk-benefit basis. Lamotrigine is excreted in breast milk. Mothers should be encouraged not to breast feed because the risks are unknown.

IV. **Adverse Drug Effects**

A. **Side Effects:** The most common side effects are dizziness, sedation, headache, diplopia, ataxia, and decreased coordination.

B. **Dermatological:** The side effect most likely to cause discontinuation of the drug is rash (10% incidence), which can be quite severe – Stevens-Johnson syndrome (toxic epidermal necrolysis). Rash is most likely to occur in the first 4-6 weeks.

C. **Metabolic:** Weight gain.

D. **GI:** Nausea and vomiting.

E. **Psychiatric:** Agitation, irritability anxiety, depression and mania.

V. **Drug Interactions**

A. Carbamazepine-induced enzyme induction will enhance lamotrigine metabolism, with subsequent lower levels than expected. Lamotrigine will increase the levels of carbamazepine and its metabolites.

B. Valproate will increase lamotrigine levels (as much as two times), and lamotrigine will decrease valproate levels slightly.

C. Phenobarbital-induced enzyme induction will lower lamotrigine levels.

D. Phenytoin will decrease lamotrigine levels.

E. No interaction with lithium has been reported.

F. Alcohol may enhance the side effects of lamotrigine.

G. Lamotrigine can be used with MAO inhibitors.

Topiramate (Topamax)

I. Indications

A. Open label studies suggest that it may have efficacy as a mood stabilizer in patients with bipolar disorder. One recent double-blind, placebo controlled study was discontinued, however, due to lack of efficacy.

B. Other open label clinical studies have suggested potential effectiveness of topiramate in bulimia, migraine, and post traumatic stress disorder.

II. Pharmacology

A. The mechanism of action is unknown.

B. Topiramate is not extensively metabolized and is mostly excrete unchanged in the urine.

C. Half-life: approximately 21 hours.

D. Preparations: 25, 100 and 200 mg tablets; 15 and 25 mg sprinkle capsules.

III. Clinical Guidelines

A. Non-psychiatric causes of mood disorder or mood symptoms (mania and depression), including medical disorders, medications and substances of abuse should be excluded before beginning topiramate treatment.

B. Screening laboratory exams should be ordered to monitor renal and hepatic function. In females of childbearing age, pregnancy should be excluded.

C. Topiramate is associated with appetite suppression and possible weight loss, a side effect that may be considered in a positive light by both the patient and the treating physician. Minimal hepatic metabolism may make it preferable over other anticonvulsants.

D. **Dosage and administration (adults)**

1. Initial dose: 25-50mg q hs then increase in 25-50mg increments per week up to 400 mg/day in divided doses.
2. Patients with renal impairment should take ½ the recommended dose.
3. No adjustments are necessary for the elderly based on age alone.

E. **Pregnancy and Lactation:** Pregnancy category C.

IV. Adverse Effects

A. The most common side effects are fatigue, somnolence, dizziness, nausea, anorexia, decreased concentration, ataxia, anxiety, and paresthesias.

B. The potential for appetite suppression and weight loss may be welcome side effects, since a significant number of psychotropic medications can cause weight gain.

V. Drug Interactions

A. Carbamazepine-induced enzyme induction will reduce topiramate levels.

B. When given with valproic acid, topiramate and valproic acid levels may decrease.

C. When given with phenytoin, topiramate levels were decreased and phenytoin levels were increased.

D. Concomitant use of phenobarbital can decrease topiramate levels.

E. Concomitant use of acetazolamide will increase the risk of nephrolithiasis and should be avoided.

F. Topiramate may decrease serum digoxin levels.

G. Topiramate may reduce the effectiveness of oral contraceptives by reducing estrogen availability.

Pregabalin

I. **Indications (FDA approval pending):** Pregabalin is currently under investigation for the treatment of epilepsy, neuropathic pain, generalized anxiety disorder, social phobia, and panic disorder. Recent studies indicate comparable efficacy to benzodiazepines, venlafaxine and SSRIs in the reduction of generalized anxiety.

II. **Pharmacology**

A. Pregabalin binds to calcium channels, not GABA receptors, and modulates calcium influx, resulting in anxiolytic, analgesic and anticonvulsant activity.

III. **Clinical Guidelines**

A. **Dosage and Administration.** The dosage of pregabalin in anxiety studies has ranged from 300 to 600 mg per day, usually given tid. The optimal dosage has yet to be determined.

B. **Response Time.** Time to response is likely similar to antidepressants, but some preliminary data indicates that pregabalin may have a more rapid onset of action.

C. **Adverse Drug Reactions:** Not fully established, but dizziness and drowsiness are common.

IV. **Drug Interactions:** Not established to date.

References, see page 102.

Psychostimulants

Dextroamphetamine (Dexedrine)

I. **Indications**
   A. Dextroamphetamine has been approved for the treatment of narcolepsy symptoms and Attention-Deficit Hyperactivity Disorder deficit hyperactivity disorder (ADHD). It is used in the treatment of ADHD in children and adults.
   B. Dextroamphetamine is used as an adjunct to antidepressants in patients who have had an inadequate response to antidepressants. It has also been used effectively in depressed medically ill or elderly patients who have not been able to tolerate antidepressants.

II. **Pharmacology**
   A. Dextroamphetamine is the d-isomer of amphetamine. It is a centrally acting sympathomimetic amine and causes the release of norepinephrine from neurons. At higher doses, it will also cause dopamine and serotonin release. It inhibits CNS MAO activity.
   B. Peripheral effects include increased blood pressure and pulse, respiratory stimulation, mydriasis, and weak bronchodilation.
   C. Preparations: Dextroamphetamine sulfate (Dexedrine) – 5, 10, 15 mg tabs; elixir 5 mg/5 mL; Dexedrine Spansule (sustained release) - 5, 10, 15 mg caps.
   D. **Half-Life:** 8-12 hrs

III. **Clinical Guidelines**
   A. Dextroamphetamine is a schedule II controlled substance, requiring a triplicate prescription. Dextroamphetamine has a high potential for abuse since it increases energy and productivity. Tolerance and intense psychological dependence develop.
   B. Symptoms upon discontinuation may include fatigue and depression. Chronic users can become suicidal upon abrupt cessation of the drug.
   C. **Pre-Dextroamphetamine Work-Up**
      1. Blood pressure and general cardiac status should be evaluated prior to initiating dextroamphetamine.
      2. Since dextroamphetamine can precipitate tics and Tourette's syndrome, careful screening for movement disorders should be completed prior to beginning treatment.
   D. Dextroamphetamine is contraindicated in patients with hypertension, hyperthyroidism, cardiac disease or glaucoma. It is not recommended for psychotic patients or patients with a history of substance abuse.
   E. **Dosage and Administration**
      1. **Attention-Deficit Hyperactivity Disorder:** Initial Dosage 2.5-5.0 mg bid-tid. Increase gradually in divided doses (7 am, 11 am or noon, 3 pm) until optimal response. Maximum dose approximately 1.0 mg/kg/day for children. Maximum 40 mg/day for adults. Spansule preparation can be given bid.
      2. **Depression (medically ill):** 5-20 mg/day.

3. **Narcolepsy:** 10-60 mg/day in divided doses.
4. Children under the age of 3 should not be given dextroamphetamine.

F. Weight and growth should be monitored in all children. Weight loss and growth delay are reasons to discontinue medication.

G. **Pregnancy and Lactation:** Pregnancy category C. There is an increased risk of premature delivery and low birth weight in infants born to mothers using amphetamines. Dextroamphetamine is contraindicated in pregnancy or breast feeding.

IV. Adverse Drug Reactions

A. **Side Effects:** The most common side effects are psychomotor agitation, insomnia, loss of appetite, and dry mouth. Tolerance to loss of appetite tends to develop. Effect on sleep can be reduced by making sure no drug is given after 12 pm.

B. **Cardiovascular:** Palpitations, tachycardia, increased blood pressure

C. **CNS:** Dizziness, euphoria, tremor, precipitation of tics, Tourette's syndrome, and, rarely, psychosis.

D. **GI:** Anorexia and weight loss, diarrhea, constipation.

E. **Growth inhibition:** Chronic administration of psychostimulants has been associated with growth delay in children. Growth should be monitored during treatment.

F. **Toxicity/Overdose:** Symptoms include insomnia, irritability, hostility, psychomotor agitation, psychosis with paranoid features, hypertension, tachycardia, sweating, hyperreflexia, tachypnea. At very high doses, patients can present with arrhythmias, nausea, vomiting, circulatory collapse, seizures and coma.

V. Drug Interactions

A. High blood levels of propoxyphene can enhance the CNS stimulatory effects of dextroamphetamine, causing seizures and death

B. Dextroamphetamine will enhance the activity of tricyclic and tetracyclic antidepressants, and will also potentiate their cardiovascular effects.

C. Dextroamphetamine may antagonize the effects of antihypertensives.

D. Typical antipsychotics and lithium can inhibit the CNS stimulatory effects of dextroamphetamine

E. Fatal reactions are likely if psychostimulants are given with MAOIs. Hypertensive crisis and seizures may occur. MAOIs should be discontinued for at least 14 days prior to the initiation of dextroamphetamine.

F. Dextroamphetamine will delay the absorption of the anticonvulsants ethosuximide, phenobarbital and phenytoin.

Dextroamphetamine and Amphetamine (Adderall, Adderall XR)

I. **Indications**
   A. Adderall is indicated for the treatment of Attention-Deficit and Hyperactivity Disorder (ADHD) and Narcolepsy.

II. **Pharmacology**
   A. Adderall is a combination of two closely related amphetamines and has a similar pharmacology to Dexedrine.
   B. **Preparations:** Adderall 5-, 7.5-, 10-,12.5-, 15-, 20-,30-mg tablets; Adderall XR 5-, 10-, 15-, 20-, 25-, 30-mg capsules
   C. **Dosing:** 5-10 mg/day with the average dose of 20-30 mg/day for ADHD and 5-60 mg for narcolepsy. Maximum dose is 40 mg for children and 60 mg for adults.

III. **Clinical Guidelines**
   A. Adderall is a schedule II controlled substance, requiring a triplicate prescription. Adderall has a high potential for abuse since it increases energy and productivity. Tolerance and intense psychological dependence develop.
   B. Symptoms upon discontinuation may include fatigue and depression. Chronic users can become suicidal upon abrupt cessation of the drug.
   C. **Pre-Adderall Work-Up**
      1. Blood pressure and general cardiac status should be evaluated prior to initiating dextroamphetamine.
      2. Since Adderall can precipitate tics and Tourette's syndrome, careful screening for movement disorders should be completed prior to beginning treatment.
   D. Adderall is contraindicated in patients with hypertension, hyperthyroidism, cardiac disease or glaucoma. It is not recommended for psychotic patients or patients with a history of substance abuse.
   E. Weight and growth should be monitored in all children. Weight loss and growth delay are reasons to discontinue medication.
   F. **Pregnancy and Lactation:** Pregnancy category C. There is an increased risk of premature delivery and low birth weight in infants born to mothers using amphetamines. Adderall is contraindicated in pregnancy or breast feeding.

IV. **Adverse Drug Reactions**
   A. **Side Effects:** The most common side effects are psychomotor agitation, insomnia, loss of appetite, and dry mouth. Tolerance to loss of appetite tends to develop. Effect on sleep can be reduced by making sure no drug is given after 12 pm.
   B. **Cardiovascular:** Palpitations, tachycardia, increased blood pressure
   C. **CNS:** Dizziness, euphoria, tremor, precipitation of tics, Tourette's syndrome, and, rarely, psychosis.
   D. **GI:** Anorexia and weight loss, diarrhea, constipation.
   E. **Growth inhibition:** Chronic administration of psychostimulants has been associated with growth delay in children. Growth should be monitored during treatment.

F. **Toxicity/Overdose:** Symptoms include insomnia, irritability, hostility, psychomotor agitation, psychosis with paranoid features, hypertension, tachycardia, sweating, hyperreflexia, tachypnea. At very high doses, patients can present with arrhythmias, nausea, vomiting, circulatory collapse, seizures and coma.

V. Drug Interactions

A. High blood levels of propoxyphene can enhance the CNS stimulatory effects of Adderall, causing seizures and death

B. Adderall will enhance the activity of tricyclic and tetracyclic antidepressants, and will also potentiate their cardiovascular effects.

C. Typical antipsychotics and lithium can inhibit the CNS stimulatory effects of dextroamphetamine.

D. Fatal reactions are likely if psychostimulants are given with MAOIs. Hypertensive crisis or seizures may occur. MAOIs should be discontinued for at least 14 days prior to the initiation of Adderall.

E. Adderall will delay the absorption of the anticonvulsants ethosuximide, phenobarbital and phenytoin.

Methylphenidate (Ritalin, Ritalin SR, Ritalin LA, Concerta, Metadate ER, Metadate CD, Focalin)

I. Indications

A. Methylphenidate is the most commonly used in the treatment of Attention-Deficit Hyperactivity Disorder (ADHD) in children and adults. It is also used in the treatment of narcolepsy.

B. Methylphenidate is also used for depression as an adjunct to antidepressants in patients who have an inadequate response to antidepressants. It has also been used effectively in depressed medically ill or elderly patients who have not been able to tolerate antidepressants.

II. Pharmacology

A. Methylphenidate is a CNS stimulant, which is chemically related to amphetamine. Methylphenidate is metabolized by hydroxylation and then renally excreted.

B. **Preparations:** 5, 10, 20 mg tabs; sustained release 20 mg tabs; LA 20, 30 and 40 mg capsules. The sustained release tablet should be swallowed whole and not crushed or chewed. Concerta comes in 18 and 36 mg extended release tablets. Metadate CD 20 mg capsules. Metadate ER 10- and 20-mg tabs. Focalin 2.5-, 5-, 10-mg tabs.

C. **Half-Life:** 3-4 hrs; 6-8 hrs for sustained release.

III. Clinical Guidelines

A. Methylphenidate is a schedule II controlled substance, requiring a triplicate prescription. It has a high potential for abuse. Tolerance and psychological dependence can develop.

B. Symptoms upon discontinuation may include severe fatigue and depression. Chronic users can become suicidal upon abrupt cessation of the drug.

C. **Pre-Methylphenidate Work-Up**
   1. Blood pressure and general cardiac status should be evaluated prior to initiating treatment. The cardiac risk with methylphenidate is less than that for dextroamphetamine.
   2. Leukopenia, anemia and elevated liver enzymes have been reported; therefore, baseline and periodic blood counts and liver function tests are recommended.
   3. Since methylphenidate can precipitate tics and Tourette's syndrome, careful screening for movement disorders should be completed prior to beginning treatment.

D. Patients with hypertension, seizure disorder and symptomatic cardiac disease should not take methylphenidate. Methylphenidate is not recommended for psychotic patients or patients with a history of substance abuse.

E. Weight and growth should be monitored in children. Weight loss and growth failure are reasons to discontinue medication.

F. **Dosage and Administration**
   1. **Attention-Deficit Hyperactivity Disorder:** Initiate with 5 mg bid. Increase by 5-10 mg each week until optimal response achieved. Usual dose: 10-60 mg/day (max 2.0 mg/kg/day). The initial dosage of Concerta is 18 mg/day, with an average dose of 18 -54 mg/day. Ritalin LA releases an immediate dose of methylphenidate with a second release(via enteric-coated, delayed release beads) four hours later. The recommended starting dosage of Ritalin LA is 20 mg, titrated by 10 mg per week as needed up to 60 mg/day. Focalin is th d-isomer (dexmethylphenidate) of methlphenidate and, the recommended conversion is half the dose of racemic methylphenidate.
   2. **Depression (medically ill):** 10-20 mg/day.
   3. **Augmentation of Antidepressant:** 10-40 mg/day.
   4. Safety and efficacy in children under the age of 6 has not been established.

G. **Pregnancy and Lactation:** Methylphenidate is contraindicated in pregnant or lactating women.

IV. **Adverse Drug Reactions**

A. **Side Effects:** The most common side effects are nervousness and insomnia. These can be reduced by decreasing dose.

B. **Cardiovascular:** Hypertension, tachycardia, arrhythmias

C. **CNS:** Dizziness, euphoria, tremor, headache, precipitation of tics and Tourette's syndrome and, rarely, psychosis

D. **GI:** Decreased appetite, weight loss. Case reports of elevated liver enzymes and liver failure.

E. **Hematological:** Leukopenia and anemia have been reported.

F. **Growth inhibition:** Chronic administration of psychostimulants has been associated with growth delay in children. Growth should be monitored during treatment.

G. **Toxicity/Overdose:** Symptoms include agitation, tremors, hyperreflexia, confusion, psychosis, psychomotor agitation, tachycardia, sweating and hypertension. At very high doses, patients can present with seizures, arrhythmias, and coma.

V. Drug Interactions

A. Methylphenidate may antagonize the effects of antihypertensives.

B. Methylphenidate decreases metabolism and increases level of the following medications:

1. Tricyclic and tetracyclic antidepressants.

2. Warfarin.

3. Phenytoin, phenobarbital and primidone.

4. Phenylbutazone.

C. Sudden Death: There have been recent case reports of sudden cardiac death when methylphenidate and clonidine have been used together.

Pemoline (Cylert)

Pemoline is chemically unrelated to amphetamine and its mechanism and site of action is unknown. It has pharmacological activity similar to the psychostimulants. Because of its association with life threatening hepatic failure, pemoline should not be used as first-line therapy for Attention-Deficit Hyperactivity Disorder.

I. Indications: Attention-Deficit Hyperactivity Disorder.

II. Pharmacology

A. Pemoline is metabolized by the liver and excreted renally. Fifty percent of the drug is excreted unchanged.

B. Preparations: 18.75, 37.5, 75 mg tablets; 37.5 chewable tablets.

C. Half-Life: 12 hrs.

III. Clinical Guidelines

A. Cylert has reduced abuse potential compared to other psychostimulants, but psychological dependence is still possible.

B. Pre-Pemoline Work-Up: Liver function tests and CBC should be ordered prior to beginning pemoline. Pemoline is contraindicated if liver function tests are abnormal or if there is a history of liver disease. Since pemoline can precipitate tics and Tourette's syndrome, careful evaluation of patients for movement disorders should be completed prior to beginning treatment. Pemoline is not recommended for psychotic patients or patients with a history of substance abuse.

C. Dosage and Administration: Initial dosage, 18.75-37.5 mg/day (8 am) Increase weekly by 18.75 mg/day until optimal response is achieved. **Maximum dose:** 3 mg/kg/day or 112.5 mg/day. Safety and efficacy in children under the age of 6 has not been established.

D. Weight and growth should be monitored in all children. Weight loss and growth delay are reasons to discontinue medication.

E. Liver function should be monitored and serum ALT levels should be determined at baseline, and every two weeks thereafter. Pemoline should be discontinued if ALT levels increase $\geq$2 times the upper limit of normal.

F. Therapeutic Response: 3-4 weeks.

G. Pregnancy and Lactation: Pregnancy Category B.

IV. Adverse Drug Reactions

A. **Side Effects:** The most common side effect is insomnia. It may resolve over time; however, dose reduction may be necessary.

B. **Hepatic:** Liver enzymes, and hepatic failure may occur. If biweekly monitoring reveals elevated liver enzymes, the drug should be discontinued.

C. **CNS:** Tremor, headache, irritability, precipitation of tics and Tourette's syndrome, decreased seizure threshold and, rarely, psychosis

D. **GI:** Loss of appetite and weight loss, which tends to be transient and usually resolves after the first few months of treatment.

E. Minimal effect on cardiovascular status occurs, particularly in comparison to Dexedrine and methylphenidate.

F. **Toxicity/Overdose:** Symptoms include nausea and vomiting, psychomotor agitation, tremor, hyperreflexia, sweating, headache, tachycardia, hypertension, confusion, hallucinations.

V. Drug Interactions. Decreased seizure threshold has been reported when pemoline is given with anticonvulsants.

Modafinil (Provigil)

I. **Indications:** Excessive Daytime Sleepiness associated with Narcolepsy. Some evidence exists for the effectiveness of modafinil (300 mg q am) for ADHD.

II. Pharmacology

A. Modafinil is metabolized by the liver (3A4 enzyme). 3A4 inhibitors or inducers may affect the metabolism of modafinil.

B. **Preparations:** 100 and 200 mg tablets.

C. Absorption is delayed by food.

D. **Half-Life:** 15 hrs.

III. Clinical Guidelines

A. Modafinil is generally well tolerated, with little effect on nighttime sleep. It has less side effects and less abuse potential than amphetamine-like stimulants.

B. Limited data suggests that modafinil may be useful in antidepressant augmentation.

C. **Dosage and Administration:** Initial dosage is 200 mg/day (8 AM). Elderly and patients with hepatic impairment require lower dose. Some patients may benefit from a mid-afternoon dose (100-200 mg). The maximum recommended daily dose is 400 mg/day.

D. **Pregnancy and Lactation:** Pregnancy Category C.

IV. Adverse Drug Reactions

A. **Side Effects:** The most common side effects are headache, nausea, diarrhea, and anorexia. Anxiety, nervousness, and insomnia have been reported but are less frequent compared to methylphenidate.

B. **Toxicity/Overdose:** Symptoms include nausea/diarrhea, palpitations, tremor, sleep disturbance, irritability, aggressiveness, and confusion.

V. Drug Interactions. Potential interactions exist with inducers, substrates, or inhibitors of 3A4 hepatic enzyme. Other potential interactions may exist with the 2D6 and 2C19, enzymes. Use with monoamine oxidase inhibitors should be avoided.

Atomoxetine (Strattera)

I. **Indications:** Attention-Deficit Hyperactivity Disorder.

II. **Pharmacology**
   A. Atomoxetine is a newly approved medication that works via presynaptic norepinephrine transporter inhibition with subsequent enhancement of noradrenergic function. Atomoxetine is not considered a psychostimulant and is not a controlled substance.
   B. **Metabolism:** Atomoxetine is metabolized via the CYP2D6 enzyme.
   C. **Half-Life:** Approximately 4 hours.
   D. **Preparations:** 10, 18, 25, 40, and 60 mg capsules.
   E. **Dosage:**
      1. In children (<70 kg) the dose should be initiated at 0.5 mg/kg and increased to target a dose of 1.2 mg/kg/day. The dose should not exceed 1.4 mg/kg or 100 mg/day, whichever is less.
      2. In adults (>70 kg), initial dose is 40 mg/day, which is increased to 80 mg/day. Dose can be increased to 100 mg/day after 2-4 weeks. The dose should not exceed 100 mg.
      3. The dose can be given in the morning or divided between morning and late afternoon/early evening.

III. **Clinical Guidelines**
   A. Dividing the dose may reduce some side effects.
   B. Dose reductions are necessary in the presence of moderate hepatic insufficiency.
   C. Atomoxetine should not be used within 2 weeks of discontinuation os a MAO inhibitor.
   D. Atomoxetine should be avoided in patients with narrow angle glaucoma and, it should be used with caution in patients with tachycardia, hypertension or cardiovascular disease.
   E. Atomoxetine can be discontinued without taper.
   F. **Pregnancy and Lactation:** Pregnancy Category C.

IV. **Adverse Drug Reactions**
   A. **Cardiovascular:** Increased blood pressure and heart rate (similar to those seen with conventional psychostimulants).
   B. **Gastrointestinal:** Anorexia, weight loss, nausea, abdominal pain.
   C. **Miscellaneous:** Fatigue, dry mouth, constipation, urinary hesitancy and erectile dysfunction.

V. **Drug Interactions:** Individuals with decreased activity of the CYP2D6 enzyme or who are taking CYP2D6 inhibitors (eg, fluoxetine, paroxetine) will have significantly greater plasma levels (fivefold) and the drug will have a longer half-life (24 hours).

References, see page 102.

Substance Dependence

Management of Substance Dependence

I. **Clinical Guidelines for the Management of Substance Dependence**

A. **Alcohol Dependence/Withdrawal:** Prolonged use of large amounts of alcohol leads to dependence and withdrawal upon discontinuation. If untreated, withdrawal can be fatal in cases where a patient develops delirium tremens and subsequent electrolyte abnormalities or cardiac arrhythmias. Benzodiazepines, such as lorazepam and chlordiazepoxide, are used to prevent withdrawal symptoms.

B. **Alcohol Relapse:** Disulfiram and naltrexone are used to help prevent relapse once a patient has been detoxified. These agents in conjunction should be used with a behavior modification program, such as Alcoholics Anonymous, in order to yield maximum benefit.

C. **Opioid Dependence/Withdrawal:** Opioid withdrawal can lead to severe symptoms and discomfort. Typical signs and symptoms of opioid withdrawal include nausea, emesis, stomach cramps, diarrhea, sweating, rhinorrhea, anxiety, muscle cramps, bone pain, and severe craving. Detoxification with methadone can alleviate the withdrawal syndrome. Clonidine is also helpful in reduction of withdrawal, but is not as effective as methadone. Adjunctive prochlorperazine (5-10 mg PO/IM q 6-8hr prn) for nausea/emesis; dicyclomine (20 mg PO q6hr.) for stomach cramps/diarrhea; ibuprofen (600 mg po q6hr prn) for muscle/bone pain; and methocarbamol (500-750 mg q6hr prn) can help during the initial days of detoxification.

D. **Nicotine Dependence:** Sustained release of bupropion has been approved for smoking cessation. Up to 50% of patients taking bupropion will achieve abstinence from tobacco after 12 weeks of treatment. This rate is twice the rate of placebo. Success of bupropion is increased by combining bupropion with a smoking cessation program.

E. **Sedative/Hypnotic Withdrawal:** Marked withdrawal symptoms can occur with abrupt discontinuation of sedative/hypnotic medications.

F. **Psychostimulant Abstinence Syndrome:** Discontinuation of psychostimulants such as amphetamines, methylphenidate, and cocaine can produce fatigue, depression, hypersomnia, and irritability. Treatment usually consists of supportive care. Benzodiazepines can be used to treat irritability.

Buprenorphine (Subutex, Suboxone)

Category: Synthetic opioid.
Mechanism: Buprenorphine is a partial agonist at the mu-opioid receptor and an antagonist at the kappa-opioid receptor.
Indications: Treatment of opioid dependence.
Preparations:
Suboxone: Tablets contain 2 mg of buprenorphine with 0.5 mg of naloxone, or tablets contain 8 mg of buprenorphine with 2 mg of naloxone.
Subutex: 2 mg or 8 mg tablets of buprenorphine alone.
Dosage:

Induction: To avoid precipitating withdrawal, Subutex should be used for induction when signs of withdrawal are present. Patients may be given Subutex, 8 mg, on day one and 16 mg of Subutex on day two. On day three and thereafter, Suboxone at a dosage of 16 mg per day is recommended.
Maintenance: Suboxone is preferred for maintenance because it contains naloxone. The recommended target dose of Suboxone is 16 mg per day. This should be accomplished by increasing the dosage by 2-4 mg per day, titrated to suppress opioid withdrawal symptoms. The range is between 4-24 mg per day.

Half-life: 37 hours for buprenorphine; 1.1 hours for naloxone.
Adverse Drug Reactions:

A. Respiratory/CNS depression can occur with buprenorphine, especially if used intravenously. The risk of respiratory depression, including possible death, is increased if buprenorphine is combined with alcohol, benzodiazepines or other CNS depressants. Caution should be used in patients with compromised respiratory function (eg, COPD, hypercapnea, cor pulmonale).
B. Buprenorphine produces opioid dependence, characterized by withdrawal if the drug is abruptly discontinued. The naloxone in Suboxone can produce marked opioid withdrawal if used intravenously or sublingually by opioid dependent patients.
C. Buprenorphine may cause hepatocellular injury, and cases of hepatic failure, hepatic encephalopathy and other hepatic disease have been reported. Liver enzymes should be measured at baseline and periodically during treatment.
D. Allergic reactions characterized by rashes, hives, and pruritis may occur. Bronchospasm, angioneurotic edema and anaphylactic shock have been seen. Hypersensitivity to naloxone is a contraindication to Suboxone.

Drug Interactions

A. CYP3A4 inhibitors, such as azole antifungals and protease inhibitors, increase the plasma levels of buprenorphine, and a decrease in the dosage of Subutex or Suboxone may be required.

B. CYP3A4 inducers, such as carbamazepine and St. John's wort, have not been systematically studied with buprenorphine but will likely decrease plasma levels and require a higher dosage of buprenorphine.

Clinical Guidelines

A. In order to prescribe buprenorphine, clinicians will need to have specialty certification in addiction medicine and complete separate training on the treatment of opioid-dependent patients. In addition, clinicians must not treat more than 30 patients in their practice, and they should be able to refer patients for adjunct services, such as psychosocial therapy.

B. Subutex should be administered at least four hours after use of heroin or other short-acting opioids, and it should ideally be administered when early opioid withdrawal signs appear.

C. There is minimal experience with transferring patients on methadone maintenance to buprenorphine, and withdrawal symptoms may occur during induction.

D. Suboxone is preferred to Subutex for maintenance due to the inclusion of naloxone.

Clonidine (Catapres, Catapres-TTS)

Category: Antihypertensive agent.
Mechanism: Alpha-2-adrenergic receptor agonist.
Indications: Used for opioid withdrawal. It may also be used adjunctively for other withdrawal syndromes, such as alcohol or sedative/hypnotic withdrawal, to dampen noradrenergic symptoms.
Preparations: 0.1, 0.2, 0.3 mg tablets; clonidine TTS patch - 2.5 mg/ 3.5 cm. (0.1 mg/day), 5.0 mg/ 7.0 cm(0.2 mg/day), 7.5 mg/ 10.5 cm (0.3 mg/day).
Dosage:

Opioid withdrawal: 0.1-0.2 mg po bid-qid with 0.1 mg q4hr prn (max 2.4 mg/day) or use a TTS patch along with po prn.

Methadone withdrawal: 0.1-0.2 mg PO bid-tid.

Half Life: 12-16 hr.
Adverse Drug Reactions: Hypotension, sedation, and dizziness may be severe. Fatigue, dry mouth, nausea, constipation, sexual dysfunction, insomnia, anxiety, depression, photophobia, rash, and weight gain may occur.
Drug-Drug Interactions

A. Potentiates the sedation with alcohol, barbiturates, and other sedative/hypnotics.

B. TCAs inhibit the hypotensive effects of clonidine.

C. Antihypertensive agents increase the hypotensive effects of clonidine.

Clinical Guidelines: Clonidine reduces the autonomic signs of opioid withdrawal. It is less effective for craving. The abrupt cessation of clonidine can lead to rebound hypertension, which can be fatal in rare instances. Clonidine should be tapered gradually over several days when discontinuing use. Use caution in patients with a history of cardiac disease or Raynaud's Syndrome.

Disulfiram (Antabuse)

Category: Aldehyde dehydrogenase inhibitor.
Mechanism: Leads to elevated levels of acetaldehyde with subsequent toxic effects.
Indications: Alcohol dependence.
Preparations: 250, 500 mg tablets.
Dosage: 250-500 mg qhs.
Half-life: 60-120 hr.
Adverse Drug Reactions:

A. Sedation, fatigue, headaches, acne, impotence, rash, metallic aftertaste, and irritability are relatively common, but usually disappear during the first few weeks of treatment.
B. Hepatotoxic effects can occur, and disulfiram should not be used in patients with preexisting liver disease.
C. Peripheral neuropathy, optic neuritis, and psychosis are rare complications of treatment.
D. If alcohol is consumed, patients will usually experience flushing, headache, nausea, vomiting, dyspnea, thirst, diaphoresis, hypotension, palpitations, chest pain, anxiety, blurred vision, and confusion. In severe cases, respiratory depression, arrhythmias, heart failure, seizures, and death may follow. Treatment of a disulfiram-alcohol interaction consists of supportive therapy. The disulfiram-alcohol reaction may occur for up to 14 days after discontinuing disulfiram.

Drug Interactions:

A. Isoniazid may cause ataxia with mental status changes.
B. Metronidazole may precipitate psychosis.
C. Disulfiram may increase levels of: diazepam, paraldehyde, phenytoin, tricyclic antidepressants, anticoagulants, barbiturates, benzodiazepines, or anticoagulants.

Clinical Guidelines

A. The combination of disulfiram with an alcohol recovery program decreases the risk of relapse. Patients must be motivated to stop drinking, otherwise, they usually stop taking the drug or drink while taking it.
B. A risk of severe alcohol reaction remains for two weeks after the last dose of disulfiram. Use caution in patients with a history of renal or hepatic disease, CNS disorder, hypothyroidism, or over age 50. Baseline liver function tests and an ethanol level are recommended.
C. Periodic monitoring of liver function tests is advised. Warn patients about dietary and over the counter preparations that may contain alcohol. Disulfiram is contraindicated in patients with severe cardiovascular or pulmonary disease.

Methadone (Dolophine)

Category: Synthetic opioid.
Mechanism: Opioid receptor agonist.
Indications: Detoxification and maintenance treatment of opioid addiction. Methadone can only be prescribed in a federally approved treatment center. The

drug may be continued if the patient is hospitalized for another reason.
Preparations: 5, 10, 40 mg tablets; 5 mg/5 mL solution, 10 mg/5 mL solution, 10 mg/mL solution. (PO); 10 mg/mL solution. (IV, IM)
Dosage:

Detoxification: Short-term use (21 days maximum). Initial dosage, 10-20 mg po on the first day. Increase by 5-10 mg per day over the next few days, up to 40 mg per day in a single or divided dosage. Maintain at this dosage for 2-5 days and then decrease by 5 mg qod.

Maintenance: Treatment with methadone after 21 days is considered maintenance. A dosage of 60-80 mg is usually effective in preventing relapse.

Half-life: 24-36 hr.
Adverse Drug Reactions:

A. Methadone produces tolerance along with physiological and psychological dependence. Tolerance to the euphoric effects may lead to overdose. Overdose can lead to respiratory and cardiovascular depression, coma, and death.
B. The most common adverse reactions include sedation, nausea, emesis, dizziness, sweating, constipation, euphoria or dysphoria, dry mouth, urinary retention, and depression.

Drug Interactions:

A. CNS Depressants can potentiate the effects of alcohol, sedative/hypnotics, other narcotics, general anesthetics, tricyclic antidepressants.
B. Desipramine may increase desipramine plasma concentrations.
C. Carbamazepine may lower plasma levels of methadone.
D. **MAOIs:** The combination of an MAOI and the opiates meperidine and fentanyl have led to fatalities.

Clinical Guidelines

A. Use caution in patients with a history of respiratory disease, hepatic or renal abnormalities, seizure disorder, or head injury.
B. Women who conceive while on methadone should continue taking the drug; however, the newborn will require medical care for withdrawal symptoms.

Naltrexone (ReVia)

Category: Opioid antagonist.
Mechanism: Antagonist of opioid receptors.
Indications: Alcohol dependence (reduce craving), opioid dependence (blocks euphoric effects of alcohol).
Preparations: 50 mg tablets.

Long-acting IM preparation is under development (150-300 mg q 4 weeks).

Dosage:

Alcohol craving: 50 mg/day.

Opioid abuse: Start with 25 mg on first day; then 50 mg/day.

Half-life: 13 hrs (including active metabolite)
Adverse Drug Reactions

A. Naltrexone may precipitate acute opiate withdrawal in patients who are still using opiates. Nausea is the most common adverse effect, which is minimized by starting with 25 mg Qod or administering with food. Other adverse effects include insomnia, headache, anxiety, fatigue, dizziness, weight loss, and joint and muscle pain.

B. Naltrexone may cause hepatocellular injury when given in excessive dosages. It is contraindicated in patients with significant liver disease. Liver enzymes should be monitored.

Drug Interactions

A. Patients who are currently using opioids will experience withdrawal due to the antagonist effect of naltrexone. If continued opioid use is suspected, a naloxone challenge may be used, and the patient is observed for signs of opiate withdrawal. Patients should be opioid free for at least 14 days before initiation of naltrexone.

B. Naltrexone will block the analgesic effects of opioids, and higher than average doses of analgesics may be needed for pain relief.

C. Disulfiram and naltrexone should not be combined because of the hepatotoxic potential of both of these agents.

Clinical Guidelines

A. Naltrexone decreases the euphoria associated with alcohol consumption when used in combination with an alcohol treatment program. It reduces craving, and there are fewer relapses. Naltrexone also lowers consumption of alcohol when a patient does relapse.

B. Naltrexone's utility in opiate dependent patients is more controversial. Some heroin dependent patients will attempt to use high dose of heroin in order to overcome the Mu receptor blockade. This can lead to accidental overdose and death by respiratory depression.

Bupropion (Zyban)

Category: Unicyclic aminoketone antidepressant.

Mechanism: Bupropion may work via alteration of dopaminergic and noradrenergic neurotransmission.

Indications: Smoking cessation.

Preparations: 150 mg sustained release tablets.

Dosage: 150 mg Qod for several days, then increase dosage to 150 mg bid

Half-life: 4-21 hr.

Adverse Drug Reactions

A. Most common side effects: Dry mouth, insomnia, dizziness, and arthralgias.

B. Seizures: Rate of seizures at doses up to 300 mg/day is 0.1%. Bupropion is contraindicated in patients with history of seizures, head trauma, brain tumor or who are taking medications that significantly lower seizure threshold. Avoid use in patients with anorexia or bulimia, due to possible electrolyte imbalances leading to seizures.

C. Mania: Bupropion can precipitate mania or rapid cycling and should be used with caution in patients with bipolar disorder.

D. Use caution in patients with hepatic, renal, or cardiac disease.

E. Neuropsychiatric: In depressed patients, bupropion has been associated with psychosis and confusion. These symptoms abate with reduction or discontinuation of bupropion.

F. Bupropion is not recommended during pregnancy or while breast feeding.

Drug Interactions

A. **Enzyme Inducers:** Enzyme-inducing agents, such as carbamazepine, phenobarbital, and phenytoin, may induce lower plasma bupropion levels.

B. Cimetidine may inhibit the metabolism of bupropion, leading to higher plasma levels.

Clinical Guidelines: Bupropion is generally well tolerated. Efficacy compared to nicotine patches or gum is unknown.

References, see page 102.

Cognitive Enhancers

I. **Indications:** Reversible acetylcholinesterase inhibitors are indicated for the treatment of cognitive impairment associated with early Alzheimer's disease.

II. **Pharmacology:** Cognitive impairment associated with Alzheimer's disease is thought to be secondary to deficiency of cholinergic neurotransmission. These medications inhibit cholinesterase, resulting in increased synaptic concentrations of acetylcholine. While these drugs do not alter the overall course of the disease, they can prolong functional status in demented patients early in the course while there are still sufficient numbers of cholinergic neurons present.

III. **Clinical Guidelines**

A. These medications improve cognitive performance in patients with mild to moderate dementia of the Alzheimer's type. Prior to treatment, patients should undergo a thorough medical examination to rule out treatable causes of dementia.

B. Cognitive function should be evaluated using standardized testing (ex: Mini-Mental Status Exam MMSE) prior to treatment and periodically thereafter to provide an objective measure of treatment response. Improvement of 1-2 points on the MMSE can be observed in patients with mild to moderate cognitive impairment. Mild to moderate is defined on the MMSE as a score between 10-26.

C. Clinical studies indicate that improvement is temporary. Decline often is evident by 30 weeks. The rate of decline appears to be slower with acetylcholinesterase inhibitor treatment.

D. Tacrine was the first acetylcholinesterase inhibitor, and it has largely been replaced by newer medications which do not carry the risk of hepatotoxicity.

IV. **Adverse Drug Reactions**

A. Due to increased cholinergic activity, gastric acid secretion can be increased, resulting in increased risk of ulcer development.

B. Other predictable adverse effects caused by the cholinergic mechanism of action include: nausea and vomiting, diarrhea, anorexia, weight loss, dizziness, syncope, and bradycardia. These tend to be dose related and can also be minimized by following manufacturer's guidelines regarding slow upward dose titration.

C. Cholinomimetics may reduce seizure threshold, and exacerbate obstructive pulmonary disease.

D. Tacrine is associated with liver toxicity.

Donepezil (Aricept)

Class: Piperidine.
Mechanism: Reversible selective acetylcholinesterase inhibitor.
Indications: Mild-to-moderate dementia of the Alzheimer's type. Donepezil does not have the potential for hepatotoxicity associated with tacrine.
Preparations: 5, 10 mg tablets.

Dosage:

Initial Dosage: 5 mg/day for four weeks.

Maintenance Dosage: Increase dose to 10 mg Qod after 4 weeks if tolerated.

Metabolism: Half-life is 70 hours; hepatic metabolism through CYP2D6 and 3A4 hepatic isoenzymes, followed by glucuronidation.

Side-Effect Profile: Most common are nausea, vomiting, diarrhea, insomnia, muscle cramps, fatigue and anorexia, which often resolve with continued treatment.

Clinical Guidelines: The 10-mg dose is associated with a higher incidence of side effects, but may be more effective. May cause syncope and exacerbate bradycardia; therefore, beta-blockers should be avoided or be given in a reduced dosage.

Galantamine (Reminyl)

Class: Tertiary alkaloid.

Indications: Treatment of mild-to-moderate Alzheimer's dementia.

Pharmacology

Mechanism of action: Reversible, competitive acetylcholinesterase inhibitor with subsequent enhancement of cholinergic function.

Half-life: Approximately 7 hours.

Preparations: 4, 8, and 12 mg tablets; 4 mg/ml oral solution.

Clinical Guidelines

Dosage and Administration:

The recommended starting dose is 4 mg bid, increasing to 8 mg twice a day (16 mg/day) after 4 weeks of treatment. A further increase to 12 mg twice a day (24 mg/day) may be attempted after a minimum of 4 weeks at the previous dose. The recommended therapeutic dose for most patients is 16-24 mg/day.

Pregnancy and Lactation: Pregnancy category B.

Adverse Drug Effects: Bradycardia, nausea, vomiting, diarrhea, anorexia, weight loss, dizziness, syncope. Side effects tend to be caused by the cholinergic mechanism of action and are dose related.

Drug Interactions: Since galantamine is metabolized via CYP2D6 and CYP3A4, inhibitors of either of these cytochrome enzymes will reduce galantamine clearance, such as paroxetine (2D6), erythromycin, nefazodone (3A4) and ketoconazole (both). No clinically significant effects on digoxin levels or prothrombin time (in patients receiving warfarin) has been noted.

Rivastigmine (Exelon)

Class: Phenyl Carbamate.

Mechanism: Reversible selective acetylcholinesterase inhibitor.

Indications: Mild-to-moderate dementia of the Alzheimer's type. Rivastigmine does not have the potential for hepatotoxicity associated with tacrine.

Preparations: 1.5, 3, 4.5, 6 mg tablets; 2 mg/mL oral solution

Dosage:

Initial Dosage: 1.5 mg bid, after 2 weeks increase to 3 mg bid

Maintenance Dosage: 3 mg bid may be effective. The dose can be increased if necessary to 4.5 mg bid, and then to 6 mg bid at two week intervals if required and if tolerated. May be given with food to reduce GI side effects.

Metabolism: Half-life is 1.5 hours. Rivastigmine is metabolized and eliminated by the kidneys. Because the dose is adjusted based on tolerability, adjustments in renally impaired patients are not always necessary.

Side Effects: Most common are nausea, vomiting, diarrhea, dizziness, anorexia, headache, abdominal pain, and sedation. Rivastigmine has more peripheral effects than donepezil, which may result in more gastrointestinal side effects.

Tacrine (Cognex)

Class: Acridine

Mechanism: Reversible non-specific cholinesterase inhibitor (inhibits both acetyl and butyl cholinesterase increasing occurrence of systemic side effects).

Indications: Mild-to-moderate dementia of Alzheimer's type. Tacrine can be hepatotoxic and is infrequently used.

Preparations: 10, 20, 30, 40 mg capsules.

Dosage:

Initial Dosage: 10 mg qid. After four weeks, the dose is increased to 20 mg qid. Daily dose is raised by 40 mg increments every four weeks to 120-160 mg/day.

Maintenance Dosage: 120-160 mg/day in divided doses or qid. Tacrine should be administered at least one hour before meals as food impairs absorption.

Metabolism: Half-life is 2-4 hours, extensive hepatic metabolism, principally by CYP 1A2 isoenzyme. Smoking reduces tacrine levels by induction of the CYP 1A2 isoenzyme. Women develop blood levels by 50% higher than men.

Side-Effect Profile: Elevation of serum transaminases is the most frequent side effect (30%). This appears to be reversible if tacrine is discontinued. Other side effects include nausea, vomiting, diarrhea, dizziness, agitation, anorexia, and confusion.

Clinical Guidelines: Serum liver function (ALT/SGPT) should be monitored every two weeks for the first 4 months of treatment. If elevation is three times normal, dose should be reduced. Elevations of more than five times normal, bilirubin above 3 mg/dL, hypersensitivity, or jaundice require immediate discontinuation.

Memantine (Axura, Ebixa)

Class: Dimethyladamantane

Mechanism: Memantine is an uncompetative antagonist of the N-methyl-D-aspartate receptor. It reduces glutamate mediated excitotoxicity.

Indications: Mild-to-moderate dementia of Alzheimer's type (FDA approval is pending).

Preparations: 10, 20, 30, 40 mg capsules.
Initial Dosage: 5 mg po qAM.
Maintenance Dosage: Increase at weekly intervals to 10 mg bid.
Metabolism: No dosage adjustment is required for patients over 65. In patients with moderate renal impairment, reduce dose to 5 mg bid. There are no active metabolites.
Side-Effect Profile: Memantine is fairly well tolerated. Side effects include dizziness, constipation and hallucinations in a small proportion of patients.
Clinical Guidelines: Memantine does not have the undesirable side effects associated with cholinesterase inhibitors. Cognitive improvement in patients with dementia treated with memantine is modest. Animal models suggest it may have neuroprotective benefits.
Drug Interactions: Memantine does not significantly interact with CYP450 enzymes. Drugs such as cimetidine, ranitidine, procainamide, quinidine and nicotine use the same renal cationic transport system and may increase blood levels of memantine. Coadministration of NMDA antagonists (amantadine, ketamine, dextromethorphan) should be avoided. Such combinations could result in development of psychosis. The actions of dopaminergic agonists and anticholinergic agents may be enhanced by memantine.

Antiparkinsonian Drugs

Psychiatric Side-Effect Management

I. **Indications:** Parkinsonian side effects are frequently encountered during treatment with typical antipsychotic agents and to a lesser degree with some of the atypical antipsychotics. Parkinsonian side effects includes tremor, rigidity, dystonias, and akathisia.

II. **Pharmacology**

A. Parkinsonian side effects are thought to be mediated by blockade of nigrostriatal dopamine D2 receptors. They typically occur early after initiation of treatment with dopamine antagonists.

B. Antiparkinsonian drugs fall into two major categories:

1. Anticholinergic drugs.
   a. Benztropine (Cogentin).
   b. Trihexyphenidyl (Artane).
   c. Biperiden (Akineton).
   d. Procyclidine (Kemadrin).
2. Dopamine agonists.
   a. Amantadine (Symmetrel).

III. **Clinical Guidelines**

A. Anticholinergic agents are frequently required when treating patients with mid- and high-potency typical antipsychotics.

B. For patients being treated for the first time with mid- and high-potency antipsychotics, prophylactic treatment with an antiparkinsonian is recommended to prevent unpleasant extrapyramidal side effects. Prevention of these side effects can improve compliance with antipsychotic medication. Patients who have past exposure to antipsychotic agents will frequently be able to report on the occurrence of extrapyramidal side effects, and the patient should receive anticholinergic agents.

IV. **Adverse Drug Reactions**

A. Anticholinergic agents can cause blurred vision, dry mouth, constipation, urinary retention, tachycardia and, less frequently, hyperthermia.

B. Elderly patients are more sensitive to anticholinergic agents and are at risk for developing anticholinergic induced delirium.

C. Anticholinergic are contraindicated in patients with glaucoma, prostatic hypertrophy, myasthenia gravis, duodenal or pyloric obstruction. Benztropine is the least sedating anticholinergic agent.

D. Anticholinergic intoxication can occur if drugs with strong anticholinergic effects are combined. Confusion, agitation, hallucinations, ataxia, tachycardia, blurred vision, mydriasis, increased blood pressure, hyperpyrexia, hot and dry skin, nausea and vomiting, seizures, coma, and respiratory arrest can occur.

Benztropine (Cogentin)

Category: Anticholinergic (muscarinic receptor antagonist).
Indications: Neuroleptic induced extrapyramidal symptoms.
Preparations: 0.5, 1, 2 mg tablets; 1 mg/mL soln. (IM).
Dosage:

Acute dystonia: 1-2 mg IM (max 6 mg/day).

Chronic Extrapyramidal Symptoms: 1-2 mg PO bid-tid. Perform trial off benztropine in 4 to 8 weeks to determine if continued use is necessary. Taper medication over 2 weeks.

Half-life: 3-6 hours
Side Effects: Drowsiness, dry mouth, blurred vision, nausea, weakness, confusion, constipation, urinary retention, sedation, drowsiness, depression, psychosis.
Interactions: Anticholinergics (eg, low-potency neuroleptics, tricyclics, over-the-counter sleep preparations); anticholinergic intoxication may develop.
Clinical Guidelines: Avoid using this medication with low potency neuroleptics because of additive anticholinergic effects. Benztropine is contraindicated in glaucoma, prostatic hypertrophy, myasthenia gravis, duodenal or pyloric obstruction. Benztropine is the most widely used agent for extrapyramidal symptoms.

Trihexyphenidyl (Artane)

Category: Anticholinergic (muscarinic receptor antagonist).
Indications: Neuroleptic induced extrapyramidal symptoms (Extrapyramidal symptoms).
Preparations: 2, 5 mg tablets, 5 mg capsules.
Dosage: Initially 1 mg Qod, then increase to 2 mg bid-qid (max 15 mg/day). Perform trial off trihexyphenidyl in 4 to 8 weeks to determine if continued use is necessary. Taper medication over 2 weeks when discontinuing.
Half-life: 4-6 hours
Side Effects: Drowsiness, dry mouth, blurred vision, nausea, weakness, confusion, constipation, urinary retention, sedation, drowsiness, depression, psychosis. May cause restlessness and euphoric symptoms.
Interactions: Anticholinergics (eg, low-potency neuroleptics, tricyclics, over the counter sleep preparations) may cause anticholinergic intoxication.
Clinical Guidelines: Avoid this medication with low-potency neuroleptics (additive anticholinergic effects). Trihexyphenidyl is contraindicated in glaucoma, prostatic hypertrophy, myasthenia gravis, and duodenal or pyloric obstruction.

Biperiden (Akineton)

Category: Anticholinergic (muscarinic receptor antagonist).
Indications: Neuroleptic induced extrapyramidal symptoms.
Preparations: 2 mg tablets; 5 mg/mL (IV, IM).
Dosage:

Acute dystonia: 2 mg IM. Repeat in 20 minutes, if needed.

Chronic extrapyramidal symptoms: 2 mg PO bid-tid (max 6 mg/day). Perform trial off biperiden after 4 to 8 weeks to determine if continued use is necessary. Taper medication over 2 weeks when discontinuing.

Half-life: 4–6 hours
Side Effects: Drowsiness, dry mouth, blurred vision, nausea, weakness, confusion, constipation, urinary retention, sedation, drowsiness, depression, psychosis. IV form is associated with orthostatic hypotension.
Interactions: Anticholinergics (eg, low-potency neuroleptics, tricyclics, over-the-counter sleep preparations) may cause anticholinergic intoxication.
Clinical Guidelines: Avoid using this medication with low-potency neuroleptics (additive anticholinergic effects). Biperiden is contraindicated in glaucoma, prostatic hypertrophy, myasthenia gravis, and duodenal or pyloric obstruction.

Amantadine (Symmetrel)

Category: Dopamine agonist
Indications: Neuroleptic induced extrapyramidal symptoms.
Preparations: 100 mg capsules; 50 mg/5 mL syrup.
Dosage:

Initial treatment: 100 mg bid (max 400 mg/day).
Perform trial off amantadine after 4 to 8 weeks to assess the need for continued use. Taper drug when discontinuing use.

Half-life: 24 hours, increased in elderly.
Side Effects: Nausea (common), dry mouth, blurred vision, constipation, anorexia, hypotension, dizziness, anxiety, tremor, insomnia, irritability, impaired concentration, psychosis, seizure.

Use caution in patients with a history of congestive heart failure and liver disease. Neuroleptic malignant syndrome has been reported with dose reduction or discontinuation of amantadine. Reduce dose in elderly. Contraindicated in pregnancy and lactation. Alcohol should not be used. Amantadine is contraindicated with renal disease or seizures.

Interactions:

A. Anticholinergics may rarely cause potentiation.
B. CNS stimulants may cause irritability, seizure, arrhythmia.
C. Thiazides may increase level of amantadine.
D. Sympathomimetics may cause potentiation.

Clinical Guidelines: Amantadine is associated with less memory impairment than anticholinergics. It is useful when anticholinergics must be avoided. Amantadine is less effective than anticholinergics in treatment of acute dystonias.

Diphenhydramine (Benadryl)

Category: Histamine receptor (H1) antagonist, muscarinic receptor antagonist
Indications: Neuroleptic-induced extrapyramidal symptoms (Extrapyramidal symptoms), mild insomnia.
Preparations: 25, 50 mg tablets; 25, 50 mg capsules; 10 mg/mL & 50 mg/mL soln. (IM, IV), 12.5 mg/5 mL elixir (PO).
Dosage:

Extrapyramidal symptoms: 25-50 mg PO Bid, for acute Extrapyramidal symptoms 25-50 mg IM or IV.

Half-Life: 1-4 hrs.
Side Effects: Dry mouth, dizziness, drowsiness, tremor, thickening of bronchial secretions, hypotension, decreased motor coordination, GI distress.
Interactions.

A. The major concern about concomitant medication use with diphenhydramine is the additive effect of other sedatives and other medications with anticholinergic activity.
B. Medical conditions that are sensitive to anticholinergic action such as narrow angle glaucoma and prostatic hypertrophy may worsen.
C. MAOI use can prolong and intensify anticholinergic effects. Opiate addicts commonly add antihistamines to enhance the subjective effect of the illicit drug.

Clinical Guidelines: Diphenhydramine is non-addicting and available over the counter.

References

References are available at www.ccspublishing.com

Selected DSM-IV Codes

ATTENTION-DEFICIT AND DISRUPTIVE BEHAVIOR DISORDERS

314.xx	Attention-Deficit/Hyperactivity Disorder
.01	Combined Type
.00	Predominantly Inattentive Type
.01	Predominantly Hyperactive-Impulsive Type

DEMENTIA

290.xx	Dementia of the Alzheimer's Type, With Early Onset *(also code 331.0 Alzheimer's disease on Axis III)*
.10	Uncomplicated
290.xx	Dementia of the Alzheimer's Type, With Late Onset *(also code 331.0 Alzheimer's disease on Axis III)*
.0	Uncomplicated
290.xx	Vascular Dementia
.40	Uncomplicated

MENTAL DISORDERS DUE TO A GENERAL MEDICAL CONDITION NOT ELSEWHERE CLASSIFIED

310.1	Personality Change Due to... *[Indicate the General Medical Condition]*

ALCOHOL-RELATED DISORDERS

303.90	Alcohol Dependence
305.00	Alcohol Abuse
291.8	Alcohol-Induced Mood Disorder
291.8	Alcohol-Induced Anxiety Disorder

AMPHETAMINE (OR AMPHETAMINE-LIKE)-RELATED DISORDERS

304.40	Amphetamine Dependence
305.70	Amphetamine Abuse

COCAINE-RELATED DISORDERS

304.20	Cocaine Dependence
305.60	Cocaine Abuse

OPIOID-RELATED DISORDERS

304.00	Opioid Dependence
305.50	Opioid Abuse

SEDATIVE-, HYPNOTIC-, OR ANXIOLYTIC-RELATED DISORDERS

304.10	Sedative, Hypnotic, or Anxiolytic Dependence
305.40	Sedative, Hypnotic, or Anxiolytic Abuse

POLYSUBSTANCE-RELATED DISORDER

304.80	Polysubstance Dependence

SCHIZOPHRENIA AND OTHER PSYCHOTIC DISORDERS

295.xx	Schizophrenia
.30	Paranoid Type
.10	Disorganized Type
.20	Catatonic Type
.90	Undifferentiated Type
.60	Residual Type
295.40	Schizophreniform Disorder
295.70	Schizoaffective Disorder
297.1	Delusional Disorder
298.8	Brief Psychotic Disorder
297.3	Shared Psychotic Disorder
293.xx	Psychotic Disorder Due to...
.81	With Delusions
.82	With Hallucinations
298.9	Psychotic Disorder NOS

DEPRESSIVE DISORDERS

296.xx	Major Depressive Disorder
.2x	Single Episode

.3x	Recurrent
300.4	Dysthymic Disorder
311	Depressive Disorder NOS

BIPOLAR DISORDERS

296.xx	Bipolar I Disorder,
.0x	Single Manic Episode
.40	Most Recent Episode Hypomanic
.4x	Most Recent Episode Manic
.6x	Most Recent Episode Mixed
.5x	Most Recent Episode Depressed
.7	Most Recent Episode Unspecified
296.89	Bipolar II Disorder
301.13	Cyclothymic Disorder
296.80	Bipolar Disorder NOS
293.83	Mood Disorder Due to... *[Indicate the General Medical Condition]*

ANXIETY DISORDERS

300.01	Panic Disorder Without Agoraphobia
300.21	Panic Disorder With Agoraphobia
300.22	Agoraphobia Without History of Panic Disorder
300.29	Specific Phobia
300.23	Social Phobia
300.3	Obsessive-Compulsive Disorder
309.81	Posttraumatic Stress Disorder
308.3	Acute Stress Disorder
300.02	Generalized Anxiety Disorder

EATING DISORDERS

307.1	Anorexia Nervosa
307.51	Bulimia Nervosa
307.50	Eating Disorder NOS

ADJUSTMENT DISORDERS

309.xx	Adjustment Disorder
.0	With Depressed Mood
.24	With Anxiety
.28	With Mixed Anxiety and Depressed Mood
.3	With Disturbance of Conduct
.4	With Mixed Disturbance of Emotions and Conduct
.9	Unspecified

PERSONALITY DISORDERS

301.0	Paranoid Personality Disorder
301.20	Schizoid Personality Disorder
301.22	Schizotypal Personality Disorder
301.7	Antisocial Personality Disorder
301.83	Borderline Personality Disorder
301.50	Histrionic Personality Disorder
301.81	Narcissistic Personality Disorder
301.82	Avoidant Personality Disorder
301.6	Dependent Personality Disorder
301.4	Obsessive-Compulsive Personality Disorder
301.9	Personality Disorder NOS

Index